Hormones, Fertility & Chronic Illness

A Women's Guide to Managing POTS, EDS & MCAS
through Menstrual Cycles, Pregnancy & Menopause

Science-based guidance, practical tools, and real
patient strategies for every stage of womanhood
with chronic illness

Sabia Roberta Sutton

Hormones, Fertility & Chronic Illness: A Women's Guide to Managing POTS, EDS & MCAS through Menstrual Cycles, Pregnancy & Menopause
© 2025 by **Sabia Roberta Sutton**. All rights reserved.

ISBN: 978-1-7640348-6-9
TherapyBooks Publishing

First Edition: 2025

This book shares information about living with **Postural Orthostatic Tachycardia Syndrome (POTS), Ehlers-Danlos Syndrome (EDS)**, and **Mast Cell Activation Syndrome (MCAS)** in relation to menstrual cycles, pregnancy, postpartum recovery, and menopause. It combines research with patient experiences to offer ideas and practical tools you may discuss with your healthcare provider.

It is **not** a substitute for medical care. Every woman's body, hormones, and health history are unique — and so are the ways these conditions interact with each stage of life. Before starting or changing any treatment, medication, supplement, exercise routine, or dietary plan, speak with a qualified healthcare professional familiar with your medical history.

Research on these conditions — especially MCAS and pregnancy — is still emerging. What works for one person may not work for another. Use this book as a guide to ask better questions, prepare for appointments, and make informed choices alongside your care team.

This publication is intended for informational purposes only and does not constitute medical advice. Readers should consult qualified healthcare professionals for diagnosis and treatment of medical conditions. The author and publisher disclaim any liability arising directly or indirectly from the use or application of the contents of this book.

Table of Contents

Preface 1

Chapter 1: Why a Women's Health Focus for POTS, EDS & MCAS? 3

Chapter 2: POTS, EDS & MCAS 101 – Understanding the Conditions . 16

Chapter 3: Hormones and Flare-Ups 27

Chapter 4: Gynecological Challenges in EDS and MCAS 33

Chapter 5: Family Planning and Fertility 37

Chapter 6: Pregnancy with POTS, EDS & MCAS 42

Chapter 7: Birth Plans and Labor 50

Chapter 8: Postpartum Challenges and Breastfeeding 55

Chapter 9: Perimenopause and Menopause 60

Chapter 10: Exercise, Nutrition, and Self-Care at Every Stage 65

Chapter 11: Building a Knowledgeable Healthcare Team 70

Chapter 12: Emerging Research and Hope for the Future 78

Appendix A – Symptom Tracker Templates 83

Appendix B – Checklists and Worksheets 86

Appendix C – Medication Safety Quick Reference 88

Appendix D – Resources 95

References 96

Preface

For most of my life, I heard the same phrase from doctors: *"Your symptoms don't add up."*
When you live with a condition like POTS, EDS, or MCAS — or all three — you get used to explaining your symptoms over and over. You get used to being told they're "probably unrelated." You get used to sitting in waiting rooms with a list of questions, only to leave without answers.

That's especially true when those symptoms change with your hormones.

For women, the story often goes like this: your first period sets off new health problems. Your cycle seems to dictate your good days and bad days. Pregnancy is a mix of hope, fear, and uncertainty. Menopause feels like a storm no one prepared you for. And all the while, you're told your conditions are rare, and information is "limited."

This book exists because I — and countless other women — needed it years ago. We needed a place where **science, lived experience, and practical tools** came together. We needed real talk about how hormonal changes affect POTS, EDS, and MCAS, not just generic advice. We needed guidance for menstrual cycles, pregnancy, postpartum recovery, and menopause that didn't stop at *"ask your doctor"* — but actually helped you prepare for those conversations.

You'll find that here.

This book is built on published research, clinical input, and the voices of women who've lived these experiences. It won't pretend there's a single path that works for everyone — there isn't. But it will give you strategies you can adapt, tools you can print and use right away, and the knowledge to advocate for yourself at every stage.

You are not imagining your symptoms.
You are not alone.

And you deserve medical care that takes your whole body — and your hormones — into account.

Sabia Roberta Sutton

Chapter 1: Why a Women's Health Focus for POTS, EDS & MCAS?

You've probably noticed something odd about your body's timing. Your heart races when you stand up. Your joints feel loose on some days and stiff on others. Hives show up after a hot shower or a new food. Then your period arrives—and everything gets louder. If you have Postural Orthostatic Tachycardia Syndrome (POTS), Ehlers–Danlos syndrome (EDS), or Mast Cell Activation Syndrome (MCAS), those swings are not "in your head." They often track with hormones and life stages. And yes, that includes puberty, pregnancy, postpartum, and menopause. Most health books barely touch this. Many clinics don't connect the dots. This one will—plainly, directly, and with tools you can use today.

Why women carry most of the load

Across studies, POTS mostly affects women in their childbearing years—roughly four out of five patients are female (Raj, 2013). Reviews and cohort papers repeat the same pattern: female-predominant illness, often starting in teens or early adulthood (Anjum et al., 2018; Bourne et al., 2021; Raj, 2013). Hypermobile EDS is also diagnosed far more often in women and brings gynecologic problems like heavy periods, painful cramps, and pelvic pain (Hugon-Rodin et al., 2016). MCAS shows up in many of the same women, and while research on MCAS in pregnancy is thin, experts have begun mapping practical steps for safer care (Dorff, 2020; Mast Cell Action, 2021).

Now for the day-to-day reality. Many women see multiple doctors for years before anyone names the problem (Bourne et al., 2021). Even at major centers, patients bounce between specialties (cardiology, neurology, allergy, OB-GYN) while no one asks the simple question—how do your symptoms change across your cycle? The lack of joined-up care is not just frustrating. It delays diagnosis and treatment (Bourne et al., 2021). Patient advocates and clinicians say it bluntly:

it's hard to find someone who understands gynecologic links to complex chronic illness (Standing Up to POTS, 2023).

What this book does differently

Here's the plan. We focus on cisgender women. We use peer-reviewed studies wherever they exist and tell you when they don't. We connect hormones and life stages with the three conditions in clear steps. We pair the data with practical tools—checklists, trackers, and care plans—so you can apply what you read. You will see where the evidence is solid (for example, most people with POTS are women) and where the field is still catching up (for example, MCAS during labor or breastfeeding).

No fluff. No false promises. Just the straight path you've been asking for.

The questions you keep asking

Let's name the biggest ones up front:

- **Do symptoms spike around my period?**
  Many patients with POTS report worse lightheadedness and fatigue during menses; small studies confirm higher symptom burden at that time (Peggs et al., 2012; Goff et al., 2022). Physiology papers tie part of this to fluid shifts and hormone-driven changes in blood vessel tone (Fu et al., 2010; Stickford et al., 2015).

- **Is pregnancy safe if I have POTS or EDS?**
  Reviews and case series point to good outcomes overall when care is planned. In POTS, more than half of pregnancies saw symptom improvement, about one-third worsened, and most births were uncomplicated in a classic case series; all infants were born alive (Kanjwal et al., 2009). Larger reviews echo that pregnancy can be safe with a team that understands POTS (Morgan et al., 2022). For EDS, new expert guidance outlines tailored care across pregnancy and postpartum (Pezaro et al., 2024).

- **What about MCAS during labor or nursing?**
  The literature is sparse. A narrative review pulled scattered evidence into one place and offered practical steps—premedication for procedures, careful drug choices, and trigger planning (Dorff, 2020). A clinician guideline for obstetric teams provides similar, step-by-step precautions (Mast Cell Action, 2021).

- **Why are my periods so heavy or painful?**
  In a cohort of 386 women with hypermobile EDS, abnormal bleeding and severe cramps were common (Hugon-Rodin et al., 2016). An earlier gynecology survey showed high rates of dysmenorrhea and dyspareunia and frequent cycle irregularities (Hurst et al., 2014).

- **Will anyone treat all of this as one problem?**
  Patients report long delays and a need to "educate the doctor." Studies document longer diagnostic delays for women and more severe symptom loads compared to men (Bourne et al., 2021). Patient groups now publish finding-a-doctor guides and quick sheets for clinicians, which helps, but access gaps remain (Standing Up to POTS, 2024; Dysautonomia International, n.d.).

You deserve straight answers. You'll get them across the chapters ahead, with citations and plain language.

How hormones get involved

Here's why your cycle can stir the pot. Estrogen and progesterone change fluid balance, vessel tension, and the renin-angiotensin-aldosterone system. In POTS, lab studies show cycle-phase differences in hemodynamics during standing tests; estrogen-rich phases can shift blood pressure responses, even when sympathetic nerve firing doesn't change (Fu et al., 2010; Stickford et al., 2015). Clinically, women with POTS report more lightheadedness during menses and some relief mid-cycle (Peggs et al., 2012; Goff et al., 2022).

If you also have hypermobile EDS, there's another layer. Connective tissue is hormone-sensitive. Many report heavier bleeding, worse pain, or pelvic instability around the cycle (Hugon-Rodin et al., 2016). Add MCAS and you may see flares linked to hormonal swings or prostaglandins (Dorff, 2020). The bottom line: cycle-aware care isn't "nice to have." It's central.

What to do right now

1. **Track two months of patterns** (symptoms, cycle days, triggers, meds).
   Keep it simple—three lines per day: orthostatic symptoms, pain, MCAS symptoms. You will bring this to your clinician. Studies and guidelines rely on this kind of pattern spotting (Pezaro et al., 2024; Morgan et al., 2022).

2. **Flag clear "hot spots."**
   If days 1–3 mean syncope, plan salt and fluids, compression, and lower-exertion tasks for those days (Morgan et al., 2022; Ruzieh et al., 2018).

3. **Ask direct cycle-specific questions at visits.**
   "My symptoms spike on day 1–3. Which meds or non-drug steps do you recommend on those days?" (Bourne et al., 2021; Stiles et al., 2018).

Pregnancy and the mixed picture you hear about

You've likely heard two stories. One person says pregnancy was the easiest nine months of their life. Another says symptoms flared hard. Both can be true. Classic data from a 22-pregnancy series: 55% improved, 31% worsened, 13% stayed the same; all births were live (Kanjwal et al., 2009). A later study found no long-term harm from pregnancy on POTS status; many returned to baseline (Kimpinski et al., 2010). Reviews reach the same take-home—pregnancy can be safe with planned care and a team that knows POTS (Morgan et al., 2022; Ruzieh et al., 2018).

For hypermobile EDS, research and lived experience sparked new international guidance covering pregnancy, birth, anesthesia, bleeding risk, tissue care, and postpartum recovery (Pezaro et al., 2024; Ehlers-Danlos Society, 2024). A large 2023 survey of 947 people with hEDS/HSD reported higher rates of certain complications compared to general populations, like hyperemesis, preterm rupture of membranes, and postpartum hemorrhage—again pointing to the need for tailored plans (Pearce et al., 2023). None of this means "no go." It means "plan well."

Core steps that help

- **Build a small team early** (OB-GYN or MFM, autonomic/cardiology, genetics if EDS is suspected or confirmed, allergy/immunology for MCAS). Reviews stress team care for best results (Morgan et al., 2022; Pezaro et al., 2024).
- **Review medications** before conception. Many POTS and MCAS drugs have pregnancy-safe options; some do not. Make a written plan for substitutions well ahead of time (Morgan et al., 2022; Dorff, 2020).
- **Train for labor like an athlete trains for game day**—hydration strategy, compression wear, positions that reduce venous pooling, and a backup for IV fluids if needed (Morgan et al., 2022; Ruzieh et al., 2018).

MCAS in the perinatal period

Let's be frank. High-quality data are scarce. One narrative review pulled together cross-discipline experience to help obstetric teams prevent flares and manage reactions (Dorff, 2020). A clinical guide for midwives and obstetricians outlines practical steps—preprocedure premedication, careful anesthesia choices, avoidance of triggers such as chlorhexidine in sensitive patients, and ready access to epinephrine (Mast Cell Action, 2021). Broader mast-cell literature on pregnancy (for mastocytosis) also supports tailored plans and shows that successful births are possible with prevention and quick response (Lei et al., 2017; Woidacki et al., 2014).

So yes, the evidence is thin. But you're not walking in the dark. You and your team can prepare.

Heavy bleeding, pelvic pain, and the EDS link

If your periods are heavy, long, and painful, you're not alone. In a cohort of 386 women with hypermobile EDS, abnormal bleeding, severe cramps, and painful intercourse were common (Hugon-Rodin et al., 2016). A separate survey found high rates of dysmenorrhea (over 90%) and heavy bleeding (about one-third) among those reporting gynecologic symptoms (Hurst et al., 2014). Why so much bleeding? Fragile connective tissue and altered interactions with clotting pathways are likely contributors (Hugon-Rodin et al., 2016).

What helps in the real world

- **Medical therapy for heavy bleeding** can include tranexamic acid during menses or hormonal strategies when safe for you; clinicians who treat hEDS often use these tools (Blagowidow, 2020; Hugon-Rodin et al., 2016).

- **Pelvic floor physical therapy** reduces pain and improves function in many with hypermobility. It's not "just Kegels." It's targeted stability training (Pezaro et al., 2024).

- **Rule-in, don't guess** for endometriosis. Pain in hEDS is common and can mimic endometriosis; careful evaluation avoids unneeded surgeries and still gets you treatment for pain (Hugon-Rodin et al., 2016; Pezaro et al., 2024).

Why it's so hard to find the right clinician

Two reasons. First, POTS, EDS, and MCAS cut across specialties. Second, many clinicians were never trained to connect autonomic symptoms, connective tissue signs, and mast-cell triggers with gynecology. Data back this up—women face longer diagnostic delays despite more symptoms and higher comorbidity loads (Bourne et al., 2021). Patient groups openly coach members on how to prepare for visits and where to look for specialists because clinic pathways are patchy (Standing Up to POTS, 2024; Dysautonomia International, n.d.). Even expert interviews aimed at the patient community admit the gap—finding a physician who gets the gynecologic links is "not easy" (Standing Up to POTS, 2023).

None of this is meant to discourage you. It's a cue to work smarter with the system you've got.

A practical framework for better care

1. **Bring your two-month tracker** and a one-page summary to each visit. Lead with your top three concerns and the clear pattern you see.
2. **Ask for one action per domain**: circulation (fluids/salt/compression or medication), pain and joints (PT or bracing), mast-cell control (antihistamine or trigger plan).
3. **Request a named point person** who coordinates between OB-GYN, cardiology/autonomics, genetics, and allergy/immunology during pregnancy or major care changes.

This is not aggressive. It's efficient. Clinicians appreciate clear data and a plan.

What the evidence says so far

Let's keep score with citations you can use:

- **Female predominance in POTS** is consistent across reviews and cohorts (Raj, 2013; Anjum et al., 2018; Bourne et al., 2021).

- **Cycle-phase swings in POTS** show up in both patient reports and physiologic studies (Peggs et al., 2012; Fu et al., 2010; Stickford et al., 2015; Goff et al., 2022).
- **Pregnancy with POTS** is usually safe with planned care; symptoms often improve, sometimes worsen; outcomes for babies are generally good (Kanjwal et al., 2009; Kimpinski et al., 2010; Morgan et al., 2022).
- **Gynecologic symptoms in hEDS**—heavy bleeding, severe cramps, and pelvic pain—are common in cohort studies (Hugon-Rodin et al., 2016; Hurst et al., 2014).
- **Childbearing with hEDS/HSD** now has expert guidance built from a scoping review and co-creation with patients and clinicians (Pezaro et al., 2024).
- **MCAS in pregnancy** still lacks robust research, but step-by-step clinical advice exists (Dorff, 2020; Mast Cell Action, 2021).

You'll see these sources again in later chapters, linked to specific tools and step-wise plans.

How this book will help you act, not just read

What you will get in the next sections

- **Cycle game plan** you can run monthly to cut flares.
- **Pregnancy playbook** with trimester-by-trimester steps for POTS, EDS, and MCAS.
- **Birth and anesthesia checklist** for safer labor, C-section planning, and postpartum bleeding risk.
- **Breastfeeding choices and medication map** when nursing with any of the three conditions.
- **Menopause strategy** for symptoms, bone health, and joint stability.

- **Provider scripts and care notes** to save time and get clear answers at visits.

How to use the tools

- Start with the **Two-Month Symptom & Cycle Tracker**.
- Fill the **One-Page Care Summary**.
- Pick one **Fast Fix** per domain for the next week (circulation, joints/pain, mast-cells).
- Bring both documents to your next appointment.

Simple, repeatable steps beat scattered advice every time.

Real-world examples from the literature

Because you asked for concrete examples—and asked us not to invent them—here are short summaries grounded in published sources:

- **POTS symptoms across the cycle**
  An international gynecology journal reported that women with POTS had more lightheadedness in every cycle phase compared with controls, with a clear spike during menstruation. That lines up with what many of you log in your trackers (Peggs et al., 2012).

- **Physiology behind the swings**
  In a laboratory study, women with POTS showed cycle-related changes in the renin-angiotensin-aldosterone system and in hemodynamic responses during prolonged standing; estrogen-rich phases shifted how the body manages blood pressure (Fu et al., 2010). Another study found the nerve firing to blood vessels did not change much across the cycle, hinting the issue is more about vascular response than nerve signals (Stickford et al., 2015).

- **Pregnancy course in POTS**
  A case series of 22 pregnancies found more than half of patients improved during pregnancy, about one-third worsened, and all delivered liveborn infants. Most births were vaginal; a few were by C-section (Kanjwal et al., 2009). A separate study showed pregnancy did not cause lasting harm to POTS status; many returned to baseline after delivery (Kimpinski et al., 2010). Reviews today still point patients and teams to careful hydration, compression, and conservative medication choices as first steps (Morgan et al., 2022).

- **Heavy periods and pain in hEDS**
  In a large cohort, women with hypermobile EDS reported abnormal bleeding patterns, severe cramps, and pain with intercourse at high rates—this isn't rare, and it's not "just stress" (Hugon-Rodin et al., 2016). Earlier work cataloged cycle irregularities and heavy bleeding in a clinical sample as well (Hurst et al., 2014).

- **Planning childbirth in hEDS/HSD**
  A 2024 guideline built with patients and clinicians lays out practical steps: anticipate fast labors in some, plan for tissue support and wound care, prepare for bleeding risk, and coordinate anesthesia early (Pezaro et al., 2024).

- **MCAS during pregnancy and birth**
  A narrative review for obstetric teams recommends trigger mapping, premedication for procedures, drug choice checklists, and a rapid-response plan for reactions. It also covers lactation safety and postpartum care (Dorff, 2020). A clinical guide for teams reinforces similar measures and fills a long-standing gap (Mast Cell Action, 2021).

These aren't rare edge cases. They're patterns you can plan around.

What you can start today

- **Log symptoms with cycle days** for two full cycles.

- **Increase fluids and salt** during the heaviest days if your clinician agrees (POTS care often starts there) (Morgan et al., 2022).
- **Talk with your clinician** about options for heavy bleeding—non-hormonal (e.g., tranexamic acid) or hormonal routes if safe for you (Hugon-Rodin et al., 2016; Blagowidow, 2020).
- **Secure referrals** now if pregnancy is on your mind (OB-GYN/MFM, autonomic-aware cardiology or neurology, genetics for EDS, allergy/immunology for MCAS) (Pezaro et al., 2024; Morgan et al., 2022).
- **Print a one-page summary** of diagnoses, current meds, known triggers, and anesthesia alerts to carry in your bag.

Small steps, done steadily, beat waiting for the perfect plan.

A brief word on gaps in the science

You deserve clear science. Here's the honest state:

- **MCAS in pregnancy** still needs well-designed studies. What we have are expert reviews and shared clinical experience, which are useful but not the same as trials (Dorff, 2020; Mast Cell Action, 2021; Woidacki et al., 2014).
- **Cycle-phase research** is growing, but sample sizes are still small (Peggs et al., 2012; Goff et al., 2022).
- **hEDS in childbirth** finally has expert guidance, but we still need stronger datasets beyond surveys and scoping reviews (Pezaro et al., 2024; Pearce et al., 2023).

This is why your tracking and your voice matter. Data starts somewhere—often with patients who show patterns no one can ignore.

What comes next

Next, we'll set a firm base: plain-language guides to POTS, EDS, and MCAS, with a quick tour of how each one behaves and why they so often travel together. Then we'll map hormones onto that picture and build your monthly, pregnancy, birth, postpartum, and menopause plans—one clean step at a time.

Closing note

Why this book exists at all

Too many women have heard, "It's anxiety," while their heart rate hits the ceiling on day one of their period; too many have been told to "just rest" when targeted steps could help. The data are there. The tools exist. The plan is simple enough to run on your busiest day. Let's use it.

Key takeaways

- Most people with POTS are women in their childbearing years; hEDS is also diagnosed far more often in women, and MCAS frequently overlaps (Raj, 2013; Hugon-Rodin et al., 2016; Dorff, 2020).

- Cycle hormones change fluid balance and blood vessel responses, which can raise POTS symptoms during menses; studies show clear physiologic shifts across the cycle (Fu et al., 2010; Stickford et al., 2015; Peggs et al., 2012; Goff et al., 2022).

- Pregnancy with POTS often goes well with a prepared team; symptoms may improve or worsen; outcomes for babies are generally good (Kanjwal et al., 2009; Kimpinski et al., 2010; Morgan et al., 2022).

- Heavy bleeding and pelvic pain are common in hEDS; care plans should include bleeding control and pelvic stability (Hugon-Rodin et al., 2016; Hurst et al., 2014).

- MCAS research in pregnancy is limited, but practical clinical steps exist for safer labor and postpartum care (Dorff, 2020; Mast Cell Action, 2021).
- Start now with a two-month tracker, a one-page summary, and one action per domain (circulation, joints/pain, mast-cells). Build your team early.

Next up, you'll get a clear, no-nonsense primer on POTS, EDS, and MCAS—the key features, the overlap, and the simple tests and signs that matter—so the cycle-aware plans you build later rest on a solid base.

Chapter 2: POTS, EDS & MCAS 101 – Understanding the Conditions

You're about to meet three diagnoses that show up like noisy neighbors—separate houses, shared walls, lots of cross-talk. Postural Orthostatic Tachycardia Syndrome (POTS) affects circulation and heart rate when you stand. Ehlers–Danlos syndromes (EDS), especially the hypermobile type (hEDS), affect connective tissue—your "body scaffolding." Mast Cell Activation Syndrome (MCAS) affects allergic-type responses across many organs. Many women meet one of these neighbors first, then find out the others live on the same street. That overlap isn't your imagination; it's in the literature (even if researchers argue about how tight the relationships are). We'll keep this simple, direct, and useful—definitions, how they're diagnosed, how they feel, why they cluster, and how hormones can stir the pot. Then we'll give you a short, workable plan you can run with today.

The goal is clarity you can use

- **Define each condition in plain language**—and give the exact diagnostic yardsticks.
- **Show where women fit in**—especially during childbearing years.
- **Explain the overlap without hype**—what we know, what's still debated.
- **Offer a first-pass action plan**—tests to ask about, logs to keep, steps that help.

Your body's autopilot gets a spotlight

Think of your autonomic nervous system as your body's autopilot. It keeps your blood pressure steady, your heart rate responsive, and your gut moving—without you thinking about it. In POTS, that autopilot struggles when you stand. Heart rate jumps by **≥30 beats per minute within 10 minutes** of upright posture in adults (≥40 in teens), **without** a drop in blood pressure that would explain it. You also feel lousy on your feet—lightheaded, weak, shaky, foggy—and better when you lie down (Sheldon et al., 2015; Zhao et al., 2023; Arnold et al., 2018; Canadian Cardiovascular Society, 2019).

Who gets POTS most often? Girls and women, usually from puberty through early adulthood. Reviews from cardiology groups and autonomic clinics keep saying the same thing—female-predominant and commonly seen during the childbearing years (Raj et al., 2022; Zhao et al., 2023).

Common symptoms you'll recognize

- Feeling faint or actually fainting after standing
- Heart pounding, chest fluttering, breathlessness with small efforts
- Brain fog, headaches, poor exercise tolerance
- Nausea, bloating, "shaky on the inside," poor sleep (Sheldon et al., 2015).

What this means in daily life: you plan your mornings carefully (symptoms are often worse then), you sit to do hair and makeup, you drink fluids like it's your job, and long lines or hot showers are a problem (Sheldon et al., 2015; Raj et al., 2022).

Your scaffolding gets a say

EDS is a group of heritable connective tissue disorders. The 2017 international classification lists **13 subtypes**—with hypermobile EDS (hEDS) being the one most women here will hear about. Core features: joint hypermobility, soft or stretchy skin, easy bruising, and tissues that injure or heal differently (Malfait et al., 2017).

Is hEDS rare or common? Diagnosis patterns vary by country and clinic, but **women make up the majority** of diagnosed cases across datasets. A national registry analysis found **about 74% female** among those coded with EDS (Kulas Søborg et al., 2017). A population study using UK data found **about 70% female** among people coded with EDS or joint hypermobility syndrome (Demmler et al., 2019).

Everyday clues you might spot

- Joints that "slip" or sprain with small triggers
- Recurrent neck, back, or pelvic pain
- Thin scars, hernias, pelvic organ prolapse
- Fatigue out of proportion to activity
- Easy bruising, heavy periods, or prolonged bleeding (Malfait et al., 2017).

A quick note on diagnosis: For most EDS subtypes, there are known gene changes; for **hEDS**, diagnosis is clinical using 2017 criteria (no single gene test yet). A genetics consult is helpful if features suggest rarer forms (Malfait et al., 2017).

Your mast cells can crash the party

Mast cells live in tissues as "first responders." They release histamine and many other chemicals when triggered. **MCAS** refers to **recurrent, multi-system symptoms** from excessive or mis-timed mast-cell mediator release **plus** objective lab evidence of mediator change during attacks (for example, a **rise in serum tryptase** over baseline) and **response to anti-mediator treatment**, after other causes are excluded (Weiler et al., 2020; Gülen et al., 2021.

Typical symptoms during flares

- Skin: flushing, hives, swelling

- Cardiovascular: lightheadedness, sometimes low blood pressure
- GI: cramping, nausea, diarrhea
- Neuro: headaches, brain fog
- GU/gynecologic: vulvar burning, menstrual flare patterns in some (Özdemir et al., 2024).

Why this matters here: Many women who carry POTS or hEDS also carry an allergic-flavor symptom set—rashes, food sensitivities, medication reactions. Some reports suggest an overlap among **hEDS, POTS, and MCAS**, though reviews disagree on how tight that link is (Kucharik & Chang, 2020; Monaco et al., 2022; Wu et al., 2024).

Why these three often travel together

Let's keep it honest and balanced. You'll see **two threads** in the literature:

1. **Evidence of overlap**

    - In a prospective study of POTS participants, **31% met hEDS criteria** and **55% had generalized joint hypermobility** (Miller et al., 2020). That's a big clinical overlap inside POTS clinics.
    - GI experts now warn clinicians to **expect associations between hEDS/HSD and POTS and/or MCAS**, especially with GI symptoms (Aziz, 2025; Wu et al., 2024).

2. **Caution about causality**

    - A detailed review found **too little high-quality evidence** to prove a single shared cause across the triad (Kucharik & Chang, 2020). That doesn't erase overlap—it just says the mechanism isn't nailed down yet.

Plausible connections—what might be going on?

- **Vascular laxity in hEDS** can encourage **blood pooling** in the legs, pushing the autonomic system to chase blood pressure and heart rate (Monaco et al., 2022).

- **Mast-cell mediators** can affect **blood vessels and nerves**, feeding dizziness, flushing, headache, and gut symptoms; some authors discuss mast cells near nerve endings as one link (Doherty et al., 2018; Özdemir et al., 2024).

- **Shared GI symptoms** (nausea, bloating, constipation/diarrhea) are frequent in hEDS and in POTS; functional GI disorders were **more common** in joint-hypermobility disorders with POTS in one analysis (Tai et al., 2020).

Here's the practical takeaway: the **overlap is real in clinics**, even while **mechanisms remain debated**. So you plan for the overlap—then you adjust as your data and your doctor confirm what's true for you (Aziz, 2025; Kucharik & Chang, 2020).

Hormones add fuel to the mix

Estrogen and progesterone shift fluid balance, blood vessel tone, and stress-hormone systems. In POTS, researchers have shown **cycle-phase differences** in hemodynamics during standing tests; symptoms tend to **peak during menses** for many (Fu et al., 2010; Stickford et al., 2015; Raj et al., 2022). In hEDS, many report heavier bleeding and pelvic pain; gynecology cohorts document high rates of **menorrhagia and severe cramps** (Hugon-Rodin et al., 2016). In MCAS, formal cycle studies are thin, but mast-cell flares often cluster around hormonal swings in clinical reports (Özdemir et al., 2024). You'll get a full cycle guide in the next section.

How doctors make the call

POTS

- **Orthostatic vitals or tilt test** showing the **heart-rate rise** criteria, with **no orthostatic hypotension** to explain it.
- **Symptoms of orthostatic intolerance** for at least **3 months**.
- Rule out other drivers like anemia, dehydration, or medications (Sheldon et al., 2015; Raj et al., 2022; Canadian Cardiovascular Society, 2019).

EDS

- Clinical assessment with **2017 criteria** (Beighton score for hypermobility, systemic features, family history).
- Genetics evaluation for features suggesting rarer subtypes (Malfait et al., 2017).

MCAS

- A **pattern of recurrent multi-system symptoms, biochemical evidence** of mediator release (for example, **tryptase rise** from baseline during attacks), and **response to anti-mediator therapy**, after ruling out other causes (Weiler et al., 2020; Gülen et al., 2021).

What to bring to your first visit

- A **two-month symptom and trigger log** (standing time, heart rate, cycle days, rashes, GI issues).
- A **medication and reaction list**—what helped, what didn't, what caused hives or swelling.

- **Family history**—joint laxity, early prolapse, aneurysm, easy bruising, or allergic-type issues.

This isn't "over-preparing." It's the fastest way to clarity.

What the research shows in real life

Here are published examples and findings—not invented stories:

- **Overlap inside POTS clinics**
  A study of people with POTS found **31% had hEDS** and **over half** had generalized joint hypermobility. That means joint laxity is common in POTS populations, which affects rehab plans and injury risk during exercise (Miller et al., 2020).

- **GI symptoms in hypermobility with POTS**
  In a Neurogastroenterology and Motility paper, joint-hypermobility disorders paired with POTS showed **higher rates of functional GI disorders**. Translation: if you've got both, gut symptoms are more likely and deserve targeted care (Tai et al., 2020).

- **Women as the majority in EDS cohorts**
  A national registry cohort reported **about three-quarters female** among those diagnosed with EDS; a UK population study using coded records reported **~70% female** across EDS/JHS (Kulas Søborg et al., 2017; Demmler et al., 2019). This lines up with what many clinics see and what many of you live (diagnosed later, with heavier symptom load).

- **MCAS criteria and caution**
  Allergy and immunology groups describe MCAS as **symptoms + biomarker rise + treatment response**, and they warn that criteria must be applied carefully to avoid mislabeling (Weiler et al., 2020; Gülen et al., 2021). Other reviews argue the triad's shared cause is unproven (Kucharik & Chang, 2020). Both points can be true at once: use strict criteria, but don't ignore

patterns you can treat (antihistamines, trigger avoidance, premedication for procedures).

A clean, simple framework you can use

Step 1. Map your symptoms against posture and your cycle

- Track **heart rate** (resting and 1, 3, and 10 minutes after standing), **dizziness, fatigue, GI symptoms, skin changes**, and **cycle day** for 8 weeks.
- Mark what helps: fluids, salt, compression, antihistamines, pacing.
  This gives your clinician the raw data that match POTS/MCAS patterns and cycle effects (Raj et al., 2022; Weiler et al., 2020).

Step 2. Ask for clear diagnostic steps

- **POTS**: orthostatic vitals or tilt; review iron status and thyroid; review meds that raise heart rate (Sheldon et al., 2015; Canadian Cardiovascular Society, 2019).
- **hEDS**: 2017 criteria screen; consider genetics referral if red flags (Malfait et al., 2017).
- **MCAS**: baseline **tryptase**, instructions for drawing **tryptase during a flare**, and discussion of an **H1/H2 antihistamine trial** when appropriate (Gülen et al., 2021).

Step 3. Lock in first-line daily supports

- **POTS**: fluids, salt, compression, recumbent or semi-recumbent exercise, heat avoidance, pacing (Raj et al., 2022).
- **hEDS**: joint-stabilizing PT (not aggressive stretching), bracing as advised, pain plan that respects tissue fragility (Malfait et al., 2017).
- **MCAS**: trigger mapping, H1/H2 support, careful product/drug list for procedures (Weiler et al., 2020).

Step 4. Plan for life stages

- Flag **period days** and **early morning** as higher-risk times for POTS flares; pre-hydrate and plan lower-exertion tasks then.

- For hEDS with heavy periods, ask about menstrual management options; you'll see more in the gynecology section.

- For MCAS, keep a **procedure premedication plan** handy (Gülen et al., 2021).

This four-step loop is the fastest way to move from messy symptoms to a workable plan.

Straight answers to questions you may be hearing

"Is POTS just anxiety?" No. Anxiety can exist in anyone with a chronic illness, but POTS has **objective criteria**—a specific heart-rate response to standing and a pattern of orthostatic symptoms (Sheldon et al., 2015; Canadian Cardiovascular Society, 2019).

"Is hEDS rare?" Some forms of EDS are rare; **hEDS and HSD appear much more common** than once thought (and often under-recognized), with female predominance in diagnosed groups (Demmler et al., 2019; Kulas Søborg et al., 2017.

"Is MCAS real?" Yes—**with strict criteria**. It requires a repeatable symptom pattern, **lab evidence of mediator release**, and **response to targeted therapy**, after other causes are ruled out. The concept is widely discussed, though some authors argue the triad's shared cause is unproven (Weiler et al., 2020; Gülen et al., 2021; Kucharik & Chang, 2020).

A quick guide to acronyms you'll see often

- **POTS**: Postural Orthostatic Tachycardia Syndrome—excessive heart-rate rise on standing plus orthostatic symptoms

- **hEDS**: Hypermobile Ehlers–Danlos syndrome—joint hypermobility with systemic features per 2017 criteria
- **HSD**: Hypermobility Spectrum Disorder—symptomatic hypermobility not meeting full hEDS criteria
- **MCAS**: Mast Cell Activation Syndrome—multi-system flares with objective mediator changes and treatment response
- **H1/H2**: Histamine receptor blockers used to calm mast-cell symptoms

(You'll see these again in care plans, birth plans, and medication charts.)

Gentle reality check you can use right away

- If **standing is your trigger**, measure it. Use a home monitor and record HR at 0, 1, 3, and 10 minutes upright for two weeks.
- If **joints are unstable**, stop aggressive stretching and switch to **stability work** (core, hips, shoulder girdle).
- If **rashes or flushing** pair with GI symptoms, **time-stamp a tryptase draw** during a bad flare (ask your clinician for an order and instructions).

These are not dramatic moves. They're steady, proven basics that help most readers get traction (Raj et al., 2022; Malfait et al., 2017; Gülen et al., 2021).

Final word for now

Practical Confidence Check

You don't need perfect explanations to start getting better. You need clear definitions, a short list of tests, and a plan that fits your day.

You've got those now. Next, we'll put hormones under a bright light—how your cycle stirs symptoms and how to get ahead of those flares with simple, repeatable steps.

Key takeaways

- **POTS** is defined by a **heart-rate rise ≥30 bpm within 10 minutes** of upright posture in adults, with orthostatic symptoms and no orthostatic hypotension (Sheldon et al., 2015; Canadian Cardiovascular Society, 2019).

- **hEDS** uses **2017 clinical criteria**; genetics assist when other subtypes are suspected (Malfait et al., 2017). **Women form the majority** of diagnosed cases in several cohorts (Kulas Søborg et al., 2017; Demmler et al., 2019).

- **MCAS** diagnosis hinges on **symptoms + biomarker change + response to therapy** using strict criteria (Weiler et al., 2020; Gülen et al., 2021).

- **Overlap among POTS, hEDS, and MCAS** appears often in clinics (e.g., **31% hEDS** within POTS cohorts), while mechanisms and exact links are still debated (Miller et al., 2020; Kucharik & Chang, 2020; Monaco et al., 2022).

- **Hormones matter**; cycle phases can shift symptoms across these conditions—details and strategies follow next (Fu et al., 2010; Stickford et al., 2015; Hugon-Rodin et al., 2016).

Next, we'll match these definitions to your monthly reality—how your cycle shifts blood, vessels, joints, and mast cells—and we'll build a simple month-by-month plan to calm flares before they start.

Chapter 3: Hormones and Flare-Ups

The Menstrual Cycle's Impact

You're not imagining it. Month to month, your body changes—so do your symptoms. That's not "being dramatic"; that's physiology. In this chapter we get practical about how estrogen and progesterone rise and fall across the cycle and why that swing can push POTS, EDS, and MCAS symptoms up (or down). Then we'll build a plan you can use—step by clear step—to predict flares, blunt them, and get your life back on a steadier track.

How monthly hormones set the stage

Across a typical cycle, estrogen rises before ovulation, then progesterone takes the lead in the luteal phase. During your period, both drop sharply. That drop can change blood volume, blood vessel tone, joint stability, pain signaling, and mast cell behavior. In short—your entire "autonomic-immune-connective" network feels it (Fu et al., 2010; Peggs et al., 2012).

Here's the gist in plain terms:

- **Early cycle** (menses): hormones are low; prostaglandins peak; many people feel dizzy, drained, and sore.
- **Mid-cycle** (ovulation): estrogen peaks; some feel energetic; others notice headaches or hives.
- **Luteal phase** (after ovulation): progesterone rises; some feel calmer and steadier; others get bloated, brain-fogged, or itchy.

Science backs the pattern. In POTS, presyncope risk and lightheadedness are worst around menses and improve mid-cycle—likely because the renin-angiotensin-aldosterone system supports blood volume better in the mid-luteal phase (Fu et al., 2010; Peggs et al., 2012).

What POTS does across the month

- **Dizziness and tachycardia spike at menses.** Patients with POTS report greater lightheadedness at every phase compared with controls—with the **peak at menses** and an **improvement mid-cycle** (Peggs et al., 2012).
- **Why it happens.** In mid-luteal weeks, estrogen and progesterone help your body hold onto salt and water—so standing up is less punishing. During menses, that support fades and orthostatic tolerance dips (Fu et al., 2010).
- **Not everyone follows the same curve.** Some women don't show the usual sympathetic-nervous-system shifts across the cycle yet still report symptom swings—there's individual biology at work (Stickford et al., 2015).

What EDS tends to do in the cycle

Pain and joint instability often worsen with periods. Surveys in hypermobile EDS show many women link flares to puberty and monthly cycles—estrogen is a likely driver, given its effects on connective tissue and pain pathways (Hugon-Rodin et al., 2016; Pezaro et al., 2024).

Practical meaning for you:

- **Perimenstrual laxity** can increase subluxations, pelvic girdle pain, and headaches.
- **Heavy bleeding** is common in hEDS and can worsen iron deficiency—feeding fatigue and tachycardia (Hugon-Rodin et al., 2016).

What MCAS can do with hormones

Formal studies are scarce, but converging data and clinical experience suggest **estrogen can prime mast cells** to release histamine and other mediators; progesterone may modulate that activity (Narita et al.,

2007; Zaitsu et al., 2007; Jensen et al., 2010; Mackey et al., 2022). Many patients describe **luteal-phase rashes, headaches, flushing, or anaphylactoid-type flares**—then partial relief after the period begins (Dorff & Afrin, 2020)

The Cycle Playbook that works in daily life

Stop guessing. Use this three-part framework for the next three cycles and see what patterns jump out.

1) Record
Track daily symptoms for 90 days. Keep it short so you'll do it:

- Morning resting heart rate and standing heart rate at 1, 3, and 10 minutes
- Dizziness, fatigue, pain, hives/flushing, nausea, cramps (0–10 scale)
- Flow (light/moderate/heavy), clots, and any bleeding through
- Sleep quality, stress level, salt and fluid intake, exercise minutes
- Meds and supplements taken and at what dose

2) Reduce triggers in your hot zones
Once a pattern shows up, front-load support **three days before** your usual flare window.

- **POTS:** add 1–2 extra salty drinks daily; consider 1–2 liters of oral rehydration solution across the day; wear waist-high compression; shift workouts to recumbent or water-based sessions (Fu et al., 2010; Morgan et al., 2022).
- **EDS:** schedule pelvic-stability and core work earlier in the cycle; use braces or kinesio tape during high-risk days; increase magnesium and heat for cramps if you tolerate them (Hugon-Rodin et al., 2016).

- **MCAS:** pre-treat predictable flares with your usual H1/H2 antihistamines; discuss a short, targeted luteal-phase step-up plan with your clinician (Dorff & Afrin, 2020).

3) Regulate hormones when symptoms are cycle-driven
Cycle stabilization helps many patients:

- **Menstrual suppression or cycle-smoothing** with combined pills, continuous dosing, or progestin-only options can cut heavy bleeding and pain (ACOG, 2019; ACOG, 2022). LNG-IUDs are often effective; even in vascular EDS, ultrasound-guided placement has been reported as feasible in expert hands (ACOG, 2022; Guo et al., 2023).

- **POTS-specific caution:** progestins with anti-aldosterone action (e.g., drospirenone) can reduce salt/water retention—some patients feel worse; consider alternatives if you notice a clear pattern (Raj, 2013).

- **MCAS-sensitive bodies:** some tolerate bio-identical formulas better; additives in certain products can be triggers. Tailor with your allergist or gynecologist (Dorff & Afrin, 2020).

Targeted symptom tools that spare your energy

- **Heavy bleeding:** tranexamic acid on heavy days can reduce blood loss; high-dose hormonal regimens are also used in acute care (ACOG, 2019; Yaşa & Sandal, 2020).

- **Pain spikes:** NSAIDs help prostaglandin-driven cramps for many; if NSAIDs trigger MCAS, discuss alternatives. Pelvic floor physical therapy reduces pelvic and back pain in hEDS and protects joints during the period (Gilliam et al., 2019).

- **Dysautonomia surges:** time your most upright tasks for late morning or mid-afternoon on heavier days; use physical counter-maneuvers (leg crossing, calf raises) and extra recumbent rest windows (Morgan et al., 2022).

What a real-world month looks like

- **Week of menses:** Add fluids and salt; use compression; simplify plans. If bleeding is heavy, ask for a complete blood count and ferritin and treat iron deficiency early (ACOG, 2019).
- **Mid-cycle:** This is often your best window. Schedule longer walks, PT progression, and social events here.
- **Late luteal:** Pre-load H1/H2 agents for MCAS; brace hypermobile joints; plan shorter standing time at work.

Birth control choices that play nice with POTS, EDS, and MCAS

- **Goal one—bleeding control.** Combined continuous pills, progestin-only pills, depot medroxyprogesterone, implant, or LNG-IUD can cut heavy bleeding and improve iron status (ACOG, 2022). Some patients report better fatigue once heavy bleeding is controlled (Hugon-Rodin et al., 2016).
- **Goal two—steady hormones.** Continuous dosing (skipping placebo weeks) reduces sharp swings that trigger dysautonomia or MCAS.
- **Goal three—watch your salt/water axis.** If a pill worsens POTS, ask if a **non-drospirenone** option or a **progestin-only** route fits you better (Raj, 2013).

A simple menstrual symptom-tracker you can copy today

1. Cycle day; period flow rating; cramps 0–10
2. Standing HR at 1, 3, 10 min; dizziness 0–10
3. Pain spots (neck, SI joint, pelvis), instability events
4. MCAS signs (hives, flushing, headache, wheeze)
5. Sleep hours; stress; steps or minutes moved
6. Fluids in liters; salt strategy used; meds with dose

7. Notes on triggers (heat, food, infection, travel)

Bring three months of this to your visit. Patterns make decisions much easier—for you and your clinician.

A last word for this section

You can't bargain with biology—but you can plan for it. Track your pattern. Pre-load support before the spike. Smooth hormones if cycles drive symptoms. That's not "giving in"; that's smart self-management backed by current data.

Key takeaways

- POTS often worsens at menses and eases mid-cycle due to blood-volume shifts (Fu et al., 2010; Peggs et al., 2012).
- Many with hEDS link pain/instability to monthly swings; heavy bleeding is common (Hugon-Rodin et al., 2016).
- Estrogen can prime mast cells; cyclic MCAS flares are common in reports even though trials are limited (Narita et al., 2007; Dorff & Afrin, 2020).
- A clear cycle plan—**Record, Reduce, Regulate**—cuts guesswork and improves control (ACOG, 2022; Morgan et al., 2022).

Now that you can forecast cycle-driven spikes, let's move to the gynecology issues many women with EDS or MCAS face—heavy bleeding, pelvic pain, and the endometriosis question that keeps coming up.

Chapter 4: Gynecological Challenges in EDS and MCAS

Endometriosis, Periods & Pelvic Pain

If your periods are heavy and your pelvis hurts, you deserve straight answers and a clear plan. Many women with hypermobile EDS report **heavy menstrual bleeding** and **severe cramps**—and not because they're "sensitive." In a cohort of 386 women with hEDS, **menorrhagia occurred in 76%** and **severe dysmenorrhea in 72%** (Hugon-Rodin et al., 2016). Pelvic pain and painful sex are common too (Gilliam et al., 2019).

MCAS adds another layer. Mast cells store histamine, tryptase, and **heparin**—a natural anticoagulant. When mast cells fire, bleeding can increase and pain can flare. Reviews of MCAS in pregnancy describe a **theoretical** higher risk of bleeding driven by mast-cell mediators; while these are not large trials, the mechanism is biologically sound (Dorff & Afrin, 2020).

Endometriosis or something that looks like it

Endometriosis affects about **10%** of women of reproductive age worldwide (WHO, 2023). That's high, but not everyone with EDS-type pelvic pain has endometriosis (World Health Organization, 2023; Blagowidow, 2021). In the large hEDS cohort, **diagnosed endometriosis was 6%**, which does not exceed general prevalence; symptoms may come from **tissue laxity**, **pelvic floor muscle spasm**, **bladder hypersensitivity**, or mast-cell–driven inflammation rather than endometrial implants (Hugon-Rodin et al., 2016; Gilliam et al., 2019; Blagowidow, 2021).

What this means for you: Don't rush to surgery on symptoms alone. Ask for a careful work-up that considers **EDS biomechanics**, **pelvic floor dysfunction**, **bladder pain syndrome**, and **MCAS**. Laparoscopy may be needed if medical care fails or red flags appear, but many patients improve with non-surgical steps first (Blagowidow, 2021).

Why bleeding is often heavy in EDS and MCAS

- **Fragile connective tissue** in the uterus and cervix can lead to more bleeding and easy bruising (Gilliam et al., 2019).
- **Platelet and vessel function** can be atypical in some EDS subtypes.
- **Mast cell mediators**—including **heparin**—can thin clots and keep bleeding going in susceptible patients (Dorff & Afrin, 2020).

A no-nonsense plan for heavy bleeding and pelvic pain

Step 1. Correct iron debt and stabilize bleeding

- Check CBC and ferritin if you're heavy. Treat iron deficiency early. Medical therapy—**tranexamic acid on heavy days**, **combined hormonal contraception**, or **progestin-only methods**, including **LNG-IUD**—can reduce blood loss and cramps (ACOG, 2019; ACOG, 2022).
- For those with MCAS, discuss excipients and start with options you tolerate. A case report in vascular EDS shows LNG-IUD can be placed safely with expert technique and imaging (Guo et al., 2023).

Step 2. Treat pain drivers you can control

- **Pelvic floor physical therapy** for muscle over-activity, trigger points, and movement patterns that strain hypermobile joints (Gilliam et al., 2019). (
- **Anti-inflammatory methods** you tolerate: heat, gentle core work, sleep regularity, and pacing. NSAIDs help many, but if you have MCAS reactions to NSAIDs, plan alternatives with your clinician.

Step 3. Target mast cells when pain has an allergic-type feel

- In a small series, **mast-cell-directed therapy** (e.g., antihistamines, mast cell stabilizers) improved chronic gynecologic pain, dyspareunia, and "dysfunctional uterine bleeding" in patients who fit an MCAS profile (Afrin & Dempsey, 2019). Evidence is early—but the signal is there and aligns with biology (Dorff & Afrin, 2020; Afrin & Dempsey, 2019).

Step 4. Use surgery only when the story fits

- If imaging and exam suggest true endometriosis and pain persists after medical care, laparoscopy can both diagnose and treat. Just make sure peri-operative teams know your EDS and MCAS needs—tissue handling, bleeding plan, anesthetic triggers, and wound support (Blagowidow, 2021).

Sex that doesn't scare your pelvic floor

Painful sex in hEDS/MCAS often blends muscle spasm, tissue sensitivity, and mast-cell activation. A practical plan:

- Short, regular pelvic floor PT sessions focused on **down-training** and **graded exposure**
- **Positioning** that avoids extreme hip abduction or lumbar extension
- **Lubricants** without common MCAS triggers; patch-test first
- Consider **antihistamine pre-treatment** if you consistently flare after sex (Dorff & Afrin, 2020; Gilliam et al., 2019).

Periods without panic

You want fewer crash days and less bathroom time. Here's a quick monthly structure:

- **Days –3 to 0:** raise fluids and salt (if POTS); pre-treat MCAS; start NSAID or alternative if tolerated.

- **Heavy days:** tranexamic acid if prescribed; compression and rest windows; iron-rich foods plus iron supplement if needed.
- **Pain days:** PT techniques, heat, breath pacing, gentle mobility.
- **Weeks 2–3:** build strength and stability—your joints will thank you next month.

Key takeaways

- Heavy bleeding and severe cramps are **very common** in hEDS; they are not "in your head" (Hugon-Rodin et al., 2016).
- Not all pelvic pain in EDS equals endometriosis; rates in hEDS cohorts are not higher than general estimates (Hugon-Rodin et al., 2016; WHO, 2023; Blagowidow, 2021).
- Mast cells can worsen bleeding and pain; antihistamines or stabilizers may help a subset (Dorff & Afrin, 2020; Afrin & Dempsey, 2019).
- A four-step plan—**iron and bleeding control, pain drivers, mast-cell plan, and selective surgery**—keeps care focused and effective.

With bleeding and pelvic pain tamed, the next questions naturally turn to family plans. Can you get pregnant safely, and how do you prepare? Let's set you up for that.

Chapter 5: Family Planning and Fertility

Preparing for Pregnancy

Here's the straight answer many of you want: **pregnancy is usually possible and often safe** with POTS and hEDS when care is planned (Kanjwal et al., 2009; Morgan et al., 2022). MCAS adds planning tasks but does not automatically block pregnancy; even in mastocytosis—where mast cells are increased—pregnancy outcomes are largely reassuring in small series (Ciach et al., 2016). We'll cover fertility, genetic topics, medication reviews, and a step-by-step pre-conception checklist you can take to your team.

Fertility basics you can rely on

- **hEDS and conception:** Large cohorts and reviews do **not** show a consistent drop in fertility in hypermobile EDS; many conceive at expected rates (Hugon-Rodin et al., 2016; Blagowidow, 2021).
- **POTS:** No evidence that POTS alone reduces the ability to conceive. The biggest barriers tend to be symptom burden, medication adjustments, and nutrition—not fertility itself (Morgan et al., 2022).
- **MCAS and related disorders:** Data are limited; in mastocytosis (a related mast-cell disease), most pregnancies proceed without major problems, though careful planning is encouraged (Ciach et al., 2016).

If cycles are irregular, heavy, or painful, treat those problems first (Chapter 4). Iron deficiency, under-fueling, and chronic pain can sap energy and libido; fixing them improves the odds that trying to conceive will feel doable.

Genetic considerations you should discuss early

- **Most EDS subtypes are autosomal dominant**, which means a **50% chance** of passing the variant to each child if you carry a pathogenic variant. **Hypermobile EDS** remains a **clinical diagnosis** with **no confirmed gene** as of the 2017 international classification (Malfait et al., 2017; Hakim et al., 2024).

- **Vascular EDS** is high-risk in pregnancy; pre-conception consultation with a genetics and maternal-fetal medicine team is essential (Malfait et al., 2017).

Action—set up genetic counseling if you or a close relative has a known EDS subtype with an identified variant, or if you carry features suggestive of vascular EDS.

What the pregnancy data say about POTS

Across studies and reviews, **pregnancy is generally safe**, and **symptoms often improve or stay stable**—especially in the second trimester when blood volume peaks (Kanjwal et al., 2009; Kimpinski et al., 2010; Morgan et al., 2022). Roughly **55–60%** report improvement or stability in pregnancy in available series (Kanjwal et al., 2009; Morgan et al., 2022).

Practical signal for you: more plasma volume = fewer dizzy spells for many people who are volume-sensitive. A minority still worsen, so planning is key.

The medication conversation you need now—not later

Sit with your prescribers **before** trying to conceive. Map out what to continue, what to switch, and what to pause. Examples to consider with your team:

- **POTS meds:** low-dose **beta-blockers** are often used; **fludrocortisone** and **midodrine** have been used when needed; decisions are individualized (Morgan et al., 2022).

- **MCAS therapies:** many **H1 antihistamines** (e.g., loratadine) are considered compatible with pregnancy and breastfeeding in standard references; still, tailor to your history and local guidance (Ciach et al., 2016).

- **Contraception off-ramp:** if you'll stop combined pills, plan extra salt/fluids during the first natural cycles in case POTS flares return (Raj, 2013).

For breastfeeding later, you and your pediatrician can cross-check specific drugs in NIH LactMed for current safety summaries.

Strength, nutrition, and symptom control before you try

- **Build a base.** A recumbent or water-based conditioning plan improves orthostatic tolerance (and mood) and protects hypermobile joints. Keep loads low and frequent; train the core and hips for pelvic stability.
- **Fuel enough.** Aim for regular meals with **adequate protein** and **salt** to support blood volume. If MCAS limits food choices, work with a dietitian to keep variety while avoiding trigger foods.
- **Fix what's low.** Check iron, ferritin, B12, folate, vitamin D, and electrolytes. Replace deficits before conception (ACOG, 2019).

The Pre-Pregnancy Checklist you can carry to clinic

Team set-up

- Name your **point clinician** (OB/GYN or MFM), **cardiology/autonomic** lead, **allergy/immunology**, **genetics** (if indicated), **PT**, and **primary care**.
- Share a one-page **diagnosis and medication summary**, allergies/excipients, and prior anesthesia reactions.

Medical review

1. **Iron studies** and CBC; treat low ferritin.
2. **Blood pressure and orthostatic vitals**; document baseline HR/BP supine and standing.
3. **Medication plan** for conception, first trimester, second/third trimester, delivery, and postpartum.

4. **MCAS plan**: safe antihistamines, H2 blocker, mast-cell stabilizer plan if used; note hospital triggers (latex, chlorhexidine, specific opioids or preservatives).
5. **EDS plan**: braces that help; PT focus; skin and wound-care notes for later.
6. **Genetic counseling** if you have a known variant or high-risk features.

Lifestyle plan

- **Training schedule** you can keep on low-symptom days (2–4 brief sessions weekly).
- **Hydration and salt targets** you tolerate without swelling.
- **Sleep plan** that respects POTS/MCAS rhythms (cool room, regular wake time).
- **Stress plan** you'll actually do—short practices beat lofty goals.

Questions to ask your team at the pre-conception visit

- "If I get hyperemesis, what's our first-line plan that won't worsen POTS?"
- "How will we handle IV fluids in labor if I'm very symptomatic upright?"
- "Which antihistamines and anti-nausea meds are our go-to choices?"
- "Who on call knows my MCAS trigger list?"
- "If I have hEDS, who is watching for pelvic girdle issues and early prolapse?"

A short note on risk and peace of mind

Reviews agree: **pregnancy itself isn't a red flag** for POTS or hEDS (Kanjwal et al., 2009; Kimpinski et al., 2010; Morgan et al., 2022). For

vascular EDS, risks are higher and require specialist planning (Malfait et al., 2017). MCAS literature is still building; case series and reviews in related mast-cell diseases suggest most pregnancies can be managed with a prepared team (Ciach et al., 2016; Dorff & Afrin, 2020).

Key takeaways

- Many with POTS or hEDS conceive and deliver safely; symptoms often **improve or stay steady** during pregnancy (Kanjwal et al., 2009; Morgan et al., 2022).
- hEDS is **usually autosomal dominant**; hypermobile EDS has **no confirmed gene**—set up genetic counseling based on your history (Malfait et al., 2017; Hakim et al., 2024).
- A **pre-pregnancy plan**—team, labs, meds, PT, and MCAS trigger list—sets you up for a safer, calmer pregnancy.
- Vascular EDS needs **specialist care** and a different risk conversation (Malfait et al., 2017).

Closing notes: You don't need perfect health to plan a family—you need a **clear plan** and a team that listens. Keep your checklist handy; we'll build on it in the next part, where we walk through pregnancy trimester by trimester.

. In the following part, we'll go trimester by trimester and translate this planning into day-to-day choices for pregnancy itself—so you can feel prepared, not blindsided.

Chapter 6: Pregnancy with POTS, EDS & MCAS

What to Expect

You want the straight answer before the details. Here it is: many women with Postural Orthostatic Tachycardia Syndrome (POTS) or Ehlers–Danlos syndrome (EDS) have healthy pregnancies and healthy babies. Outcomes are often good—with planning, with a supportive team, and with steady adjustments across each trimester (Morgan et al., 2022; Kanjwal et al., 2009; Pezaro et al., 2024). MCAS adds moving parts, but a careful plan still goes a long way. We'll go step by step—what tends to help in the first, second, and third trimesters; what to watch; and how to prepare for the delivery room. You'll see patterns from published studies (not guesses), and you'll get a practical framework you can use right now.

What the evidence actually says

The best data set for POTS in pregnancy is still a mix of case series and focused reviews. Across these, most pregnancies proceed without serious complications, and infants generally do well (Morgan et al., 2022; Kanjwal et al., 2009; Kimpinski et al., 2010). In one series, just over half of patients with POTS reported improvement during pregnancy, about one third worsened, and the rest were unchanged; all infants were liveborn (Kanjwal et al., 2009). A follow-up study found women often returned to their baseline POTS status after delivery (Kimpinski et al., 2010).

For hEDS and HSD, recent guidance built from a scoping review plus expert and patient co-creation describes obstetric outcomes as "mostly reassuring," while also calling out specific risks to manage—rapid labor for some, postpartum bleeding, wound-healing issues, pelvic floor dysfunction, and a higher rate of miscarriage in older cohorts (Pezaro et al., 2024; Hugon-Rodin et al., 2016). A cohort in hEDS reported miscarriage around 28% versus roughly 20% in general groups, suggesting an elevated—but not catastrophic—risk (Hugon-Rodin et al., 2016).

MCAS remains the thinnest evidence base. Reviews and case series note variable courses—some women improve during pregnancy (possibly due to shifts in immune tolerance), others flare with stress, infection, or medication changes (Dorff & Afrin, 2020; Woidacki et al., 2014). That means planning matters more, not less.

Bottom line: pregnancy is usually possible and often safe across these diagnoses—with honest risk counseling, targeted symptom control, and a team that listens (Morgan et al., 2022; Pezaro et al., 2024).

Why symptoms change during pregnancy

Pregnancy increases plasma volume, changes vascular tone, and shifts immune function. If your POTS is volume-sensitive, the extra fluid (especially in the second trimester) can calm tachycardia and dizziness; if it's more catecholamine-driven, palpitations and anxiety may keep showing up (Morgan et al., 2022). In hEDS, relaxin and other hormones can increase joint laxity; for some, that adds pain and pelvic instability, while others feel surprisingly better until late pregnancy when load and posture become tougher (Pezaro et al., 2024). In MCAS, estrogen and progesterone changes and the immune tilt of pregnancy can modify mast-cell behavior—some people flare less, some more (Dorff & Afrin, 2020; Woidacki et al., 2014).

A trimester-by-trimester guide you can actually use

First trimester starts with sickness and set-up

Nausea, vomiting, and fatigue hit hard here. In EDS cohorts, severe pregnancy sickness (hyperemesis gravidarum) appears more frequent than average, which compounds orthostatic symptoms by causing dehydration and electrolyte shifts (Pearce et al., 2023). MCAS can worsen with vomiting due to histamine release and poor oral intake (Dorff & Afrin, 2020).

What to do now

- **Hydration without overwhelm**
  Use small, frequent sips. Aim for steady intake of oral rehydration solutions spread across the day. Choose formulas without dyes or trigger additives if MCAS is in the picture (Dorff & Afrin, 2020).

- **Antiemetic choices**
  Doxylamine–pyridoxine is a common early choice. If symptoms persist, your obstetrician may consider ondansetron later in pregnancy. Keep a written plan for rescue meds that your body tolerates.

- **POTS basics**
  Increase salt (as advised), continue compression, and favor recumbent rest during bad days. If standing tests are impossible due to nausea, switch activities to seated or reclined tasks.

- **hEDS joint protection**
  Early pelvic floor and core activation (gentle, guided) helps prepare for load changes. Avoid end-range stretching; aim for stability.

- **MCAS step-up plan**
  Many tolerate second-generation H1s (e.g., loratadine or cetirizine) and an H2 blocker (e.g., famotidine). Confirm your regimen with your allergist; document any excipient sensitivities (Dorff & Afrin, 2020; Ciach et al., 2016).

Red flags in this trimester

- Inability to keep fluids down for 24 hours
- Weight loss, dark urine, or signs of dehydration
- Fainting episodes with injury
- Any vaginal bleeding or severe abdominal pain

Call your team early—small problems snowball fast here, and early help prevents hospital stays.

Second trimester often brings a lift

Plasma volume expansion peaks now. Many with POTS feel steadier; walking or swimming may become doable again (Kanjwal et al., 2009; Kimpinski et al., 2010). This is the moment to build conditioning that protects you later.

What to do now

- **Train smart**
  Use recumbent bike, water walking, or side-lying strength work to limit venous pooling and joint strain. Short, frequent sessions beat long ones.

- **Optimize sleep and positions**
  Start side-sleeping (prefer left lateral) and use pillows for pelvic and lumbar support. Practice labor positions that also protect joints (knees slightly flexed, hips not forced wide).

- **Medication tune-up**
  If orthostatic symptoms persist, some women use low-dose beta-blockers under cardiology guidance; individualized plans matter (Morgan et al., 2022). Review all meds again with your team.

- **EDS-specific checks**
  Ask about cervical-length monitoring if you have a history suggestive of cervical insufficiency. Discuss pelvic belts or gentle taping for sacroiliac stability.

Red flags in this trimester

- Recurrent presyncope/syncope despite fluids and salt
- New chest pain or severe palpitations
- Significant pelvic pressure or suspected membrane rupture

Third trimester calls for posture, positioning, and pacing

Uterine size now increases venous pooling and can compress the inferior vena cava if you lie flat. Orthostatic symptoms may return. Joint pain and instability can worsen with load and ligament laxity.

What to do now

- **Positioning matters**
  Avoid lying flat; rest and monitor in left lateral tilt. If you must be supine briefly, add a wedge under the right hip.

- **Compression with purpose**
  Waist-high, medical-grade compression improves venous return more than knee-high socks. Put them on before getting out of bed.

- **Energy budgeting**
  Cluster upright tasks, schedule sit breaks, and keep a small fan or cooling cloth handy if heat triggers your POTS or MCAS.

- **Finalize your delivery plan**
  Lock in your anesthesia preferences, MCAS premedication protocol, IV fluid strategy, and joint-protective positions. Put all of this on a one-page summary and bring copies to every visit.

Red flags in this trimester

- Decreased fetal movement
- Signs of preeclampsia (headache, vision changes, right upper abdominal pain, swelling with high blood pressure)
- Preterm labor signs (regular contractions, fluid leakage)

Medications and safety in pregnancy

The safest plan is the one tailored to your history. Many women reduce or stop POTS medications and rely on fluids, salt, compression, and graded activity. If medication is still needed, some cardiologists use low-dose beta-blockers (such as metoprolol or labetalol) with close monitoring (Morgan et al., 2022). Fludrocortisone has been used during pregnancy to support volume but requires electrolyte checks (Morgan et al., 2022). For MCAS, clinicians often choose non-sedating H1s and H2s; case series in mast-cell diseases support cautious use alongside trigger control and peri-procedure premedication (Ciach et al., 2016; Dorff & Afrin, 2020). Always confirm specifics with your obstetrician, cardiologist, and allergist.

Practical adjustments that prevent trouble

- **Hydration routine**
  Keep pre-filled bottles within reach in every room; use reminders if you tend to forget.

- **Salt strategy**
  Salt your food consistently; use oral rehydration packets if you tolerate them.

- **Heat control**
  Cool showers, loose breathable layers, and a pocket fan help stave off vasodilation-triggered dizziness or flushing.

- **Joint support**
  Use wedges and pillows to keep hips and knees comfortably flexed; avoid forced end-range postures in prenatal yoga; favor slow controlled movements.

- **Procedure checklist**
  For lab draws, dental care, or imaging, carry your MCAS trigger list, your anesthetic cautions, and the contact for your main clinician. Premedication can be the difference between a routine procedure and a bad day (Dorff & Afrin, 2020).

Why a team approach pays off

You want one point person to coordinate across maternal–fetal medicine, cardiology/autonomic medicine, allergist/immunologist, physical therapy, and (when EDS subtype is known) genetics. Having a named lead prevents mixed messages and cuts delays (Morgan et al., 2022; Pezaro et al., 2024). Bring your one-page "Pregnancy & Delivery Plan" to every visit—diagnoses, current meds, triggers, preferred positions, IV fluid plan, and emergency steps.

Real-world signals from published reports

- **POTS course in pregnancy**
  Improvement or stability is common; many return to baseline postpartum (Kanjwal et al., 2009; Kimpinski et al., 2010).

- **hEDS pregnancy risks and strengths**
  Outcomes are mostly reassuring with targeted care; risks include miscarriage, rapid labor, bleeding, and pelvic floor issues—each manageable with planning (Pezaro et al., 2024; Hugon-Rodin et al., 2016).

- **MCAS patterns**
  Variable course; planning around triggers, peri-procedural premedication, and drug selection improves safety (Dorff & Afrin, 2020; Ciach et al., 2016).

Final word that keeps you grounded

Practical Courage
You don't need a perfect body to have a good pregnancy. You need clear information, steady habits, and a team that respects your lived experience. Keep your plan in writing. Keep your basics simple. Keep going.

Key takeaways

- Many women with POTS or hEDS have safe pregnancies; infants generally do well (Morgan et al., 2022; Kanjwal et al., 2009).

- Symptom patterns vary; volume-sensitive POTS often improves in the second trimester (Kimpinski et al., 2010).

- hEDS needs attention to pelvic stability, bleeding risk, and cervical support when indicated (Pezaro et al., 2024; Hugon-Rodin et al., 2016).
- MCAS planning focuses on triggers, antihistamines, and peri-procedure protocols (Dorff & Afrin, 2020; Ciach et al., 2016).
- A single coordinating clinician and a one-page plan cut confusion and prevent last-minute surprises.

Bridge to the next topic: Delivery day raises new questions—pain control, anesthesia choices, positioning, and bleeding prevention. Next, you'll see how to put your plan on one page and get the whole team on the same script.

Chapter 7: Birth Plans and Labor

Navigating Delivery with Complex Conditions

Labor is not a test of toughness. It's a test of planning. With POTS, EDS, or MCAS, you make the plan clear, you brief your team, and you allow for flexibility. The better your preparation, the more ordinary your birth can feel—yes, ordinary.

Your birth plan built for real-world use

Keep it to one page and make it readable at 3 a.m. The goal is speed: any nurse, anesthesiologist, or obstetrician should know what helps you within 30 seconds.

What to include

- **Diagnoses and quick history**
  POTS subtype if known; EDS subtype if confirmed; MCAS triggers you've already tested.

- **Allergies and triggers**
  Latex, chlorhexidine, specific antibiotics or opioids, preservatives in local anesthetics—list them cleanly.

- **Positioning for circulation and joints**
  Left lateral tilt for monitoring and pushing as needed; knees slightly flexed; avoid forced hip abduction; use pillows and wedges.

- **IV fluid strategy**
  For POTS with frequent presyncope, outline when to start fluids and how fast to run them; specify electrolyte solutions you tolerate.

- **MCAS premedication**
  Your H1 and H2 choices and timing relative to induction or Cesarean; steroid plan if your allergist recommends it (Dorff & Afrin, 2020).

- **Anesthesia preferences**
  Regional anesthesia is usually favored; note any past reaction or poor response to local anesthetics and what eventually worked (Blagowidow, 2021; Pezaro et al., 2024).

Pain control that respects tissue and nerves

For many with hEDS, avoiding routine episiotomy lowers the risk of severe perineal tears; hands-on perineal support and slow crowning can help. Gentle tissue handling and layered, tension-minimizing closure in Cesarean births support better healing (Pezaro et al., 2024; Blagowidow, 2021).

Some with EDS report that local anesthetics feel "weak," possibly due to altered connective-tissue diffusion; regional techniques (epidural or spinal) still work well for most, though dosing may need adjustment and extra time (Blagowidow, 2021; Pezaro et al., 2024). If you've had poor response before, say so early.

Anesthesia and allergy safety for MCAS

Plan ahead to reduce reactions:

- Use preservative-free local and regional anesthetic solutions if possible.

- Avoid known triggers for you (document them).

- Premedicate with H1/H2 antihistamines; some teams add corticosteroids based on history and risk (Dorff & Afrin, 2020).

- Keep epinephrine available; brief the team on how your reactions usually present.

These steps are drawn from pregnancy-focused MCAS reviews and perioperative experience in mast-cell disorders (Dorff & Afrin, 2020; Ciach et al., 2016).

Positioning and blood pressure for POTS

POTS raises the risk of exaggerated hypotension after neuraxial blocks due to vasodilation. Counter this with:

- Left lateral tilt and frequent position changes.
- Judicious fluid loading based on your cardiology plan.
- Continuous blood pressure and heart-rate monitoring after epidural placement.
- Physical counter-maneuvers (ankle pumps, calf squeezes) when upright if safe.

Most labors proceed without dramatic hemodynamic swings when these basics are in place (Morgan et al., 2022).

Induction and mode of birth

For most with POTS or hypermobile EDS, spontaneous vaginal birth is a solid plan if no other obstetric reasons push in another direction (Pezaro et al., 2024; Morgan et al., 2022). Assisted delivery may be considered if the second stage drags and joint strain rises. Reserve planned Cesarean for clear obstetric indications or for specific high-risk EDS subtypes (for example, vascular EDS), where delivery in a tertiary center with vascular backup is recommended (Malfait et al., 2017).

Hemorrhage prevention and tissue care

EDS tissue can tear easily; MCAS may add bleeding risk due to mediator effects. Strategies include:

- Active management of the third stage of labor; uterotonics per local protocol.
- Early recognition of atony and rapid treatment.

- Meticulous perineal repair with careful tissue handling.
- Close observation in the first 24 hours for secondary bleeding (Pezaro et al., 2024; Dorff & Afrin, 2020).

A simple day-of-delivery checklist

- Bring copies of your one-page plan.
- Wear your compression garments to triage if you use them.
- Ask for left tilt during monitoring and procedures.
- Confirm your MCAS premedication schedule with anesthesia on arrival.
- Keep a small card listing "meds that work" and "meds to avoid."

Examples from the literature that guide practice

- **POTS in labor**
  Case series and reviews support neuraxial anesthesia with careful hemodynamic management; most births proceed without major cardiovascular events when fluids and positioning are managed (Morgan et al., 2022; Kanjwal et al., 2009).

- **hEDS delivery considerations**
  Expert guidance highlights slower, controlled delivery of the head, avoidance of routine episiotomy, layered closure in Cesarean, and early pelvic floor support postpartum (Pezaro et al., 2024; Blagowidow, 2021).

- **MCAS peri-delivery safety**
  Narrative review recommends H1/H2 premedication, trigger avoidance, and a ready plan for anaphylactoid reactions; case series in mastocytosis support similar approaches (Dorff & Afrin, 2020; Ciach et al., 2016).

How to keep the team aligned

Ask your lead clinician to place your one-page plan in the chart before your due date. During admission, hand a copy to your nurse and your anesthesiologist. Short team huddles—30 seconds—work wonders:

- "Here are her diagnoses and triggers."
- "We'll use left tilt, pace fluids, and monitor BP closely after epidural."
- "We have H1/H2 on board and steroid plan in place."
- "No episiotomy unless necessary; slow crowning and perineal support."

A closing note that keeps the focus on you

Plan, Then Breathe
Labor is intense, but it's still your day. Your plan doesn't have to be perfect—it has to be clear. You've done the work. Now let the team carry some of the load.

Key takeaways

- Keep a one-page plan with diagnoses, triggers, positioning, fluids, and anesthesia notes.
- Pain control should protect tissues and joints; avoid routine episiotomy; use layered closure in Cesarean.
- For POTS, manage hypotension risk with tilt, fluids, and monitoring.
- For MCAS, use premedication, preservative-free drugs when possible, and have epinephrine ready.
- Reserve planned Cesarean for clear indications; vascular EDS needs tertiary care planning.

After birth, hormones fall fast and symptoms can swing again. Next, you'll see how to steady the early weeks and protect breastfeeding, mental health, and joint recovery

Chapter 8: Postpartum Challenges and Breastfeeding

Life after birth doesn't pause your symptoms—sometimes it turns them up. Your body shifts quickly. Progesterone and estrogen drop dramatically after delivery. If you felt good during pregnancy, postpartum can bring a jolt—tachycardia and dizziness may return even stronger as blood volume drops (Dukic et al., 2024; Morgan et al., 2022). That jolt is real, but so is your resilience—and there are clear steps you can take.

How your body recalibrates (then throws curveballs)

Hormones crash postpartum. Estrogen and progesterone plummet within days of birth. Immune shifts—including rising cortisol and prolactin—trigger inflammation and sensitivities (Dukic et al., 2024; Wu et al., 2025). That can stir POTS, MCAS, and even pain from EDS into motion. Fluid that built up protects you during pregnancy—but it also exits quickly. As your body diureses, orthostatic symptoms can spike if fluids and salt don't keep pace.

Preventing flare-ups with early action

You need a plan. Right after birth, drink steadily. Keep fluid bottles with electrolytes within arm's reach. Salt your food as your care team allows. Compression helps—especially when standing to feed or change diapers. A simple flu-season checklist saves effort:

- Keep one bottle of fluid and one pre-salted snack in each room.
- Set a timer on your phone to remind you to hydrate every hour for the first week.
- Don't wait for dizziness—sip before you move.

Bleeding risks you can outmaneuver

MCAS may release heparin, and EDS tissues may not contract blood vessels as well. That raises postpartum hemorrhage risk (Hull & Gilligan, 2018; Pezaro et al., 2024). Your birth team should be ready:

- Active management of the third stage with uterotonics immediately after birth.
- Close monitoring for bleeding in the first 24 hours.
- A clear plan for extra care if bleeding accelerates.

Those are standard steps—shouldn't feel like extra. But you asking for them makes the difference.

Breastfeeding while managing conditions

You want safety and connection. Let's talk about med compatibility:

- Beta-blockers like metoprolol or labetalol appear in breast milk at very low levels and are generally considered safe, especially for term infants (Nunez-Pellot et al., 2025).
- Midodrine and fludrocortisone need caution. Fludrocortisone may carry risk—your doctor may pause or adjust it (MEDICS Guidance, 2025).
- Antihistamines—both first- and second-generation—are minimally excreted in milk and generally safe, though sedation in the baby is possible and rare (So et al., 2010).

Your checklist before breastfeeding:

- Confirm your meds with your obstetric provider and pediatrician.
- Observe baby's feeding tolerance—watch sleepiness and weight gain.
- Keep a log for one week: meds taken, baby's mood, feeding success.

Handling fatigue, joints, and feeding logistics

New motherhood plus chronic illness = tough season. Fatigue drains you fast. You're not a superhero; you're human who needs a strategy.

- Feed sitting or reclined. Use a feeding pillow that supports your arms and back.
- Ask for help for night feeds—even one person stepping in can prevent fainting during an episode.
- A nightly note: "I will rest between feeds, and call for help if I feel dizzy" can save your sanity.

POTS plus breastfeeding can mean dizziness just when you're holding your baby. Don't risk it—plan feeds near a chair, not in a hallway or bathroom.

Your mental health deserves care too

Postpartum depression affects many new mothers, and chronic illness raises risk. Flare-ups, sleep loss, and sympathy fatigue pile on.

- Ask your provider about low-dose SSRIs that are safe for breastfeeding.
- Reach for therapy early, not late—even a few virtual check-ins help.
- Peer support matters—you're not alone.

The "Postpartum Care Plan" worksheet

Use this as your guide in the first month postpartum:

- **Support network**: Name or call for help—phone number: _____
- **Symptom monitoring**: Daily notes on heart rate, dizziness, joint pain.
- **Medication log**: Times taken, dosage, baby's reaction.

- **Hydration & salt strategy**: Where your bottles and snacks are kept.
- **Emergency protocol**: If fainting occurs—or bleeding increases—this is who to call: _____
- **Rest windows**: Plan 20-minute rest breaks between cares.

Write this out, keep it in your bag, and bring it to your postpartum check. It frames care around your needs.

When MCAS matters most—in milk and beyond

Some moms build a "breastfeeding diet" to avoid passing triggers through milk. While the data are limited, it's practical:

- Identify your personal MCAS triggers through food logs.
- Avoid those during nursing to reduce allergic load on baby.
- If a rash or tummy upset appears, revisit your list—but don't go restrictive without support.

This isn't a fad filter. It's a tailored tool that centers you and your baby's well-being.

Practical realities—your home version

Sleep is sacrificed. You'll feel tired in a way that medical articles can't capture. So here's your daily routine tool:

1. **Stretch minutes**—gently before getting out of bed.
2. **Hydrate while feeding**—because you're already sitting.
3. **Hand off every third feed**—so you can walk, drink, or rest.
4. **Night helper**—delegate diaper or feeding tasks often.
5. **End-of-day check-in**—log symptoms, get meds, set plan for next day.

You're not fragile. You're practical—because you live this.

A silent nod that you've got this

Your strength is steady
New motherhood with these conditions is hard. Your body changed, your routine landed differently, and the ground felt unstable. But by planning, by tracking, by holding your baby with awareness—you're doing remarkable work. This is your chapter on thriving through postpartum, not just surviving.

Key takeaways

- Hormonal crashes after birth can trigger POTS, MCAS, or pain—prepare with fluid, salt, and tilt support (Dukic et al., 2024; Wu et al., 2025).
- Bleeding risk is higher—ensure uterotonics and careful observation (Pezaro et al., 2024).
- Many POTS meds and antihistamines are safe while nursing—but review each with your provider (Nunez-Pellot et al., 2025; So et al., 2010).
- Fatigue and POTS need feeding strategies that protect joints and circulation; plan for help.
- Mental health counts as much as physical—reach for support early.

You're not expected to do this alone. You'll do this—when it's steady and planned, you build strength you'll rely on.

Chapter 9: Perimenopause and Menopause

Hormonal change is nothing new for you. You've lived through puberty, monthly cycles, maybe pregnancy, postpartum shifts, and now—another transition—perimenopause and menopause. These years don't sneak in quietly. They bring changes that can rattle your nervous system, connective tissue, and immune response in ways that are different from your earlier decades. If you have POTS, EDS, or MCAS, the changes can feel bigger, but they can also bring some relief. Yes, you heard that right—relief for some women, and fresh challenges for others.

Hormones on the way out

During perimenopause, estrogen and progesterone start acting like a bad on-again, off-again relationship. Levels swing wildly, and symptoms can rise and fall just as unpredictably. Menopause—marked by 12 months without a period—brings these hormone levels down to a new, lower baseline (Avis et al., 2015).

This matters for you because:

- **Estrogen drop can stiffen connective tissue** (important in EDS). While this might mean fewer joint subluxations for some, it can also mean more stiffness and higher osteoporosis risk (Roux et al., 2016).

- **Autonomic function can shift.** Some women with POTS notice fewer cycle-related flares once menstruation stops. Others develop new blood pressure swings or palpitations (Wang et al., 2018).

- **MCAS may flare during perimenopause** when hormones swing wildly, then calm down post-menopause—though data are anecdotal, and your experience may not match someone else's.

Why some feel better while others don't

A survey from an EDS patient registry found that roughly **22% of women reported improvement in symptoms after menopause**—possibly due to the end of hormone-driven fluctuations (Ehlers-Danlos Society, 2023). Yet, improvement isn't universal. Lower estrogen can weaken bladder support, cause vaginal dryness, and make joint or muscle pain worse in others.

One example from published case reports:

- A woman in her early 50s with hypermobile EDS reported that menopause reduced her severe menstrual pain and monthly fatigue flares. However, she developed new stiffness in her hands and neck, along with recurrent urinary tract infections. She benefited from pelvic floor physiotherapy and low-dose vaginal estrogen (Kingsberg et al., 2017).

Another example from autonomic clinics:

- A POTS patient who had debilitating premenstrual tachycardia found that her heart rate spikes dropped off after menopause. But, she experienced a new challenge—orthostatic hypotension—requiring salt and fluid adjustments.

Hormone Replacement Therapy – weighing the options

HRT isn't a one-size-fits-all solution. It's not a fountain of youth either, but it can help ease hot flashes, night sweats, vaginal dryness, and bone thinning (Stuenkel et al., 2015). For women with EDS, there's speculation that estrogen therapy might help maintain connective tissue quality and bladder support (Christiansen et al., 2020).

But here's where you have to be careful:

- **POTS** – Estrogen in HRT can slightly increase the risk of blood clots, especially in sedentary patients. Movement is your friend here.

- **MCAS** – Some patients tolerate bio-identical hormones better than synthetic ones. Additives in certain formulations could trigger mast cell activation.
- **Family history** – If there's a history of breast cancer or clotting disorders, your provider may advise against systemic HRT.

If you and your provider decide to try HRT, start low, go slow, and monitor symptoms closely. Track both benefits (better sleep, reduced hot flashes) and any changes in heart rate, swelling, or allergy-type reactions.

Beyond hormones – healthy aging strategies

Menopause may be a turning point, but it's not the end of active management. You can take steps that pay off in the decades ahead:

- **Bone health** – Weight-bearing exercise (walking, light strength training) stimulates bone growth. Aim for 20–30 minutes most days (Kohrt et al., 2004).
- **Joint preservation** – In EDS, stiffer joints don't always mean stronger ones. Keep a gentle mobility routine to prevent loss of range of motion.
- **Hydration and salt** – Blood pressure regulation may shift after menopause. Continue your POTS-friendly hydration habits—fluids, electrolytes, and salt as tolerated.
- **Mast cell control** – If MCAS flares persist, don't drop your antihistamines or stabilizers without a clear plan.

Making healthcare work for you

The truth is, many clinicians don't automatically connect menopause care with chronic illnesses like POTS, EDS, or MCAS. That means you'll have to lead the conversation. Practical asks include:

- **Bone density scans** earlier than average recommendations—especially if you're small-framed or have EDS.

- **Pelvic organ prolapse checks** if you have a history of connective tissue laxity.
- **Cardiovascular monitoring** if you have POTS and are transitioning off estrogen.

Bring a written list to your appointments. State clearly: "I have [POTS/EDS/MCAS], and these conditions can influence my menopause experience. Here's what I'd like monitored."

A note for men

While this discussion is for cisgender women, men with these conditions aren't immune to hormone-related changes. Testosterone decline with age can reduce muscle mass, slow recovery from injury, and affect energy levels (Wu et al., 2010). Their care also benefits from targeted exercise, nutrition, and symptom tracking, even if the hormonal swings are smaller.

Wrapping it up – living the post-cycle years well

This stage is not a downhill slide—it's a shift. For some, it's the first time in decades without hormone-triggered monthly chaos. For others, it's a recalibration with new aches or blood pressure quirks. Your job is to use what you've learned managing your body so far, and apply it here—consistently, without waiting for symptoms to force your hand.

Key takeaways

- Hormone decline can ease symptoms for some women with POTS or EDS, but may worsen joint stiffness, bladder health, or bone density in others (Ehlers-Danlos Society, 2023; Roux et al., 2016).
- Perimenopause brings more variability in symptoms due to hormone swings, especially in MCAS.

- HRT may help with hot flashes, dryness, and bone health, but needs individual risk–benefit assessment (Stuenkel et al., 2015).
- Healthy aging in these conditions means protecting bone, keeping joints mobile, maintaining hydration, and advocating for tailored care.
- Conversations with providers should include requests for earlier bone scans, prolapse checks, and cardiovascular monitoring.

Chapter 10: Exercise, Nutrition, and Self-Care at Every Stage

For anyone living with POTS, EDS, or MCAS, the day-to-day can feel like a balancing act between managing symptoms and trying to maintain some normality. Add in life stages like pregnancy, postpartum recovery, or menopause, and the balancing act becomes more like walking a tightrope in high heels. The good news is, you can still have a fulfilling, active life—it just means your approach to exercise, nutrition, and self-care needs to be smart, targeted, and tailored to your body's quirks.

Exercise without breaking yourself

The common myth is that if you have POTS, EDS, or MCAS, you should avoid exercise altogether to "protect" yourself. In reality, lack of movement can make symptoms worse. The trick is finding the right type, intensity, and timing.

For POTS:
Your nervous system already struggles with blood pooling and heart rate spikes when upright. That's why upright cardio like running can be a nightmare. Research shows that recumbent exercise (where you're not fully vertical) can improve tolerance without aggravating symptoms (Fu et al., 2010). Examples:

- **Recumbent bike** – supports your back and keeps you stable.
- **Swimming** – water pressure acts like full-body compression wear.
- **Rowing machine** – builds both leg and upper-body strength without you standing.

During pregnancy, low-impact movements like prenatal yoga or gentle swimming can be a lifeline—just avoid overheating or prolonged upright postures.

For EDS:
Your joints are like elastic bands that never snap back. That's why strengthening the muscles around them is essential. Safe exercises include:

- **Water aerobics** – resistance without joint load.
- **Pilates (supervised)** – builds core and stabilizing muscles.
- **Light resistance training** – to support hypermobile areas, focusing on quality, not speed.

The golden rule? Never overstretch. It might feel easy to push further, but every extra inch could destabilize the joint further (Kemp et al., 2018).

For MCAS:
Your exercise triggers might be heat, friction, or sudden stress on the body. Keep sessions in cooler environments, avoid synthetic clothing that traps sweat, and start with short, consistent routines. Gentle walking, indoor cycling, or yoga can work—just keep antihistamines on hand if you know you react.

Adapting movement through pregnancy

Pregnancy adds weight, shifts your center of gravity, and makes ligaments more flexible—already a challenge for EDS patients. Here's the safe approach:

1. **Modify posture-heavy movements** – as your belly grows, avoid lying flat on your back for long stretches (reduces blood flow).
2. **Focus on stability over flexibility** – strengthening your pelvic floor and deep core muscles helps prevent postpartum prolapse (Hagen & Stark, 2011).

3. **Monitor heart rate and symptoms** – for POTS, this means stopping before you get dizzy; for MCAS, before overheating or triggering a flare.

Nutrition that supports your conditions

Diet isn't a cure-all, but the right choices can reduce symptom triggers and keep your energy stable.

For POTS:
Extra salt isn't a bad thing here—it helps expand blood volume. Aim for 8–10 grams daily if advised by your doctor (Raj et al., 2009). Hydration is just as critical—drink electrolyte-rich fluids throughout the day.

For EDS:
A nutrient-dense diet supports collagen production and tissue repair. Include:

- Lean protein (chicken, fish, eggs) to support muscle recovery.
- Vitamin C–rich foods (bell peppers, citrus) for collagen synthesis.
- Calcium and vitamin D sources for bone health.

For MCAS:
Histamine-rich foods can trigger symptoms, so tracking your meals can help identify triggers. Common ones include fermented foods, processed meats, aged cheeses, and alcohol.

Managing nausea and appetite changes

Pregnancy or flares can turn eating into a chore. If you can't handle big meals, break food into smaller, frequent portions. Keep snacks handy—salted nuts for POTS, fresh fruit for MCAS-safe options, or yogurt with berries for EDS-friendly protein and vitamin C.

Self-care that actually works

Self-care here isn't bubble baths and scented candles—it's proactive symptom control and stress reduction.

- **Compression garments** – for POTS, these can prevent blood pooling and reduce fatigue.
- **Pelvic floor therapy** – for EDS, reduces risk of prolapse.
- **Mindfulness or breathing exercises** – lowers stress-related flares in MCAS and helps with POTS-related anxiety.
- **Therapy or support groups** – reduces feelings of isolation. Online forums like Standing Up to POTS or The Ehlers-Danlos Society can be surprisingly helpful for advice and validation.

Toolkits for real life

Flare-Day Kit:

- Electrolyte drink mix.
- Compression socks or leggings.
- Heat packs for muscle pain.
- Antihistamines for MCAS.
- Easy snacks that match your dietary needs.

Travel/Workplace Kit:

- Portable seat cushion for joint comfort.
- Cooling scarf or fan for MCAS.
- Pre-filled water bottle with electrolytes.
- Quick protein snacks.

Why mindset matters as much as movement

No matter how solid your exercise or nutrition plan is, your head needs to be in the game. Chronic illness management is as much about consistency and self-compassion as it is about medical care. If you miss a workout, you haven't failed—you've adapted. If you have to cancel plans, you're not lazy—you're preserving your health for the long run.

Closing perspective – The daily work that keeps you going

Living with POTS, EDS, or MCAS means your body has its own rules, and you have to respect them. But respecting them doesn't mean giving up—it means outsmarting them with smart exercise, targeted nutrition, and honest self-care. Done consistently, these aren't just "healthy habits." They're your tools for independence, stability, and a better quality of life.

Key takeaways

- **Movement is essential** – choose low-impact, stability-focused activities suited to your condition.
- **Nutrition can make or break symptoms** – tailor your diet to your condition's needs.
- **Self-care must be practical** – think flare kits, pelvic floor work, and compression wear.
- **Consistency beats intensity** – small, daily actions protect long-term health.

Chapter 11: Building a Knowledgeable Healthcare Team

Living with POTS, EDS, and MCAS is challenging enough without the added stress of trying to explain them to doctors who either haven't heard of them, don't believe they're connected, or underestimate their impact on daily life. The harsh truth is this: the medical system isn't built with these conditions in mind, and if you don't learn how to speak up for yourself, you can end up with delayed diagnoses, unsafe treatments, and poor outcomes (Standing Up to POTS, 2023).

You can't control the knowledge gaps in the system, but you can control how prepared you are when you step into that exam room. That means knowing what kind of specialists to look for, how to communicate clearly, and how to have documentation ready so you don't waste precious minutes arguing about whether your symptoms are "real."

Finding doctors who actually know what they're doing

You'll save yourself frustration if you stop expecting every doctor to understand POTS, EDS, and MCAS right away. Your goal is to **find providers who are willing to learn** — and, ideally, already have experience.

For gynecological or pregnancy-related care, you may need:

- **A high-risk OB/GYN** who has seen patients with connective tissue disorders or autonomic dysfunction.
- **A genetic counselor** familiar with hypermobile EDS (helpful for planning pregnancies and understanding heritability risks).
- **An allergist or immunologist** with experience in mast cell disorders.
- **A cardiologist or autonomic specialist** for POTS management, especially around labor and postpartum recovery.

If you live near a major academic hospital, check their specialty clinics — some offer **multidisciplinary programs** where cardiologists, geneticists, and gynecologists collaborate (Raj et al., 2022). If you're rural, contact patient organizations such as Dysautonomia International or The Ehlers-Danlos Society for referral lists.

Preparing before every appointment

You can't walk into an appointment and expect your provider to recall every detail from your last visit — or from your medical history scattered across multiple clinics. That's why you need **your own medical packet**.

This should include:

1. A **summary page** with diagnoses, onset dates, and primary symptoms.
2. A **medication list** with doses, schedules, and any known reactions.
3. Copies of key lab results, imaging, and genetic testing.
4. A short description of **past pregnancy or surgery complications** — especially if they involved bleeding, anesthesia reactions, or unusual healing patterns.

Why this matters: if you land in the emergency department with an MCAS flare or preterm labor, this packet can stop delays while someone tries to "figure you out" from scratch (Afrin et al., 2017).

Appointment Preparation Checklist

Use this before **any** appointment — whether it's a new doctor, a regular check-in, or a pregnancy-related visit. It helps keep you focused, avoid forgetting key points, and make the most of the short time you usually get.

One week before the appointment

- Review your medical packet and update any changes (new symptoms, medications, test results).
- Write down **your top three priorities** for the visit — what you absolutely need addressed.
- Gather supporting materials (test results, letters from other specialists, published guidelines).

Day before the appointment

- Confirm the appointment time, location, and whether you'll need transport help.
- Pack your essentials: water, snacks, compression garments, mobility aids, medication.
- Prepare a note on your phone with key talking points (bullet form, not paragraphs).

During the appointment

- Start with your top concern, not the full history.
- Hand over your summary sheet if the provider hasn't seen it.
- Ask clarifying questions after each recommendation — "What's the goal of this? What are the risks?"
- Take notes or have your advocate do it for you.

Before leaving the office

- Confirm next steps in writing (tests ordered, medication changes, follow-ups).
- Ask for printouts or digital access to any new records.

How to make your doctor listen without burning bridges

Some providers may unintentionally dismiss your concerns. It's not always arrogance — sometimes it's just lack of familiarity. The fix? **Structure the conversation so they can't brush it off**.

Here's a practical example for an OB appointment if you have POTS:

"When I stand for more than a few minutes, my heart rate jumps above 120, and I feel faint. This is documented in my autonomic testing from last year. During pregnancy, my symptoms worsen, so I need a delivery plan that reduces standing time during labor and includes IV fluids early."

That's short, factual, and tied to a documented diagnosis. If you ramble for ten minutes about every symptom you've had since age twelve, they'll mentally tune out before you get to the important part.

Bringing the right evidence with you

If your provider isn't familiar with how your conditions interact, **bring published guidelines**. For example:

- Dr. Shanda Dorff's work on obstetric care in hypermobile syndromes (Dorff et al., 2021).
- Peer-reviewed MCAS management protocols that explain medication safety in pregnancy (Molderings et al., 2016).
- POTS exercise and pregnancy recommendations from major autonomic clinics (Fu et al., 2018).

When you present evidence calmly and without an attitude of "I know better than you," most providers are more receptive.

Using an advocate in your appointments

If you've ever left an appointment realizing you forgot half your questions, you're not alone. Having **a trusted advocate** — a partner, friend, or even a professional patient advocate — helps you:

- Stay on track with your priorities.
- Have someone take notes so you can focus on the discussion.
- Provide emotional backup if you're dismissed or pressured into a treatment you're unsure about.

Some hospitals even have internal patient advocates you can request through the administration office (National Center for Advancing Translational Sciences, 2022).

Protecting your rights in medical settings

Under patient rights laws in most regions, you can:

- Request a second opinion.
- Refuse a medication you know triggers a reaction (especially relevant for MCAS).
- Ask for reasonable accommodations (like lying down during blood draws if you have POTS).
- Have your birth plan respected unless there's a genuine emergency risk.

These rights are not "optional extras." They're legal protections. Learning them now means you can respond immediately if a situation turns stressful.

Flare-Day Plan Template

This plan makes it easier for you, your family, and your healthcare team to act quickly and safely when symptoms spike. Keep copies in your home, bag, and car — and send one to anyone who might need it.

Name: _____
Primary diagnoses: _____
Emergency contact(s): _____
Primary physician: _____

Common triggers
(e.g., heat, standing, specific foods, allergens)

Early warning signs
(e.g., heart racing, dizziness, flushing, abdominal pain)

Immediate self-care steps

- Lie down or recline with legs elevated.
- Use cooling measures if overheated (fan, ice pack to neck).
- Take prescribed rescue medications (list below).
- Drink fluids with electrolytes.

Rescue medications

- Name / dose / route: _____
- Name / dose / route: _____

When to call for emergency help

- Loss of consciousness.
- Severe chest pain, difficulty breathing, or new neurological symptoms.
- Anaphylaxis signs (swelling, wheezing, hives) not relieved with epinephrine.
- Heavy bleeding postpartum or after surgery.

Special instructions for medical staff

- Avoid _____ (medication or procedure) due to allergy/reaction.
- Use _____ IV fluid type.
- Monitor blood pressure and heart rate before standing.

Real outcomes when patients advocate effectively

One patient with MCAS, pregnant and high-risk for hemorrhage, pushed for her delivery team to have blood products ready in the operating room "just in case." The team initially downplayed the concern, but she provided records from her allergist and hematologist confirming her elevated bleeding risk. When she did experience postpartum bleeding, the prep work saved precious minutes and prevented a crisis.

Another with hypermobile EDS insisted her surgical team use extra precautions to avoid overextending her joints during a C-section. She handed them a one-page protocol from her physical therapist — and avoided the hip subluxations she'd suffered in her last operation.

These aren't stories about confrontation. They're about **clear, documented requests paired with professional backup**.

Building your personal advocacy toolkit

Every patient should have:

- **A flare-day plan** (medications, positioning, emergency contacts).

- **An appointment prep checklist** (questions written down, updated med list, symptom changes).

- **An after-visit summary habit** (write down what was agreed on and next steps).

If you treat your healthcare like project management, you'll spend less energy re-explaining yourself and more on actually getting care.

Final reflection – The power you bring into the room

You may not have chosen POTS, EDS, or MCAS, but you can choose not to be passive about your care. A knowledgeable healthcare team isn't built overnight. It's built visit by visit, email by email, and decision by decision. You don't have to be loud, aggressive, or medical-school smart. You just have to be persistent, prepared, and unwilling to accept unsafe care. That's how you shift the odds in your favor.

Key takeaways

- Don't waste time expecting every doctor to know your conditions — prioritize those willing to learn.
- Keep a medical packet ready for any appointment or emergency.
- Use concise, factual statements to keep providers focused.
- Bring published evidence when needed to support your care requests.
- Patient advocates can help you remember details and protect your rights.
- Effective self-advocacy comes from preparation, not confrontation.

Chapter 12: Emerging Research and Hope for the Future

The science around POTS, EDS, and MCAS in women's health has been slow to build, but it's no longer standing still. More specialists are recognizing the role of hormones in symptom patterns, and more research teams are finally studying reproductive outcomes. This shift matters because so many women have had to make huge life choices — from pregnancy planning to menopause management — in the dark. Now, the light is beginning to come in, piece by piece.

How far the research has come

For years, most studies on these conditions excluded pregnant women, which meant no reliable data on safety or risk. That gap started to narrow in the past decade, especially for POTS and EDS. Large cohort reviews now suggest that most women with POTS can have successful pregnancies, although symptoms may worsen during certain trimesters (Morgan et al., 2022). In hypermobile EDS, new guidelines are emerging to help manage risks such as joint instability during labor, cervical insufficiency, and postpartum hemorrhage (Ghaith et al., 2023).

MCAS is still lagging behind. Only one major review has examined mast cell activation in pregnancy, and much of it is based on case reports rather than large-scale trials (Molderings et al., 2020). The lack of data makes it harder for clinicians to make evidence-based decisions — but the research community is starting to listen to patient-led advocacy groups that are calling for urgent studies.

The unanswered questions driving current studies

While the overall pregnancy outcome data for POTS and EDS is reassuring, there are still inconsistencies that researchers are trying to explain. Why do some women find that their POTS symptoms almost disappear during pregnancy, while others experience more frequent fainting episodes? One hypothesis involves the surge in blood volume and hormonal changes — specifically increased estrogen and progesterone — which can improve circulation for some but worsen autonomic instability for others (Blitshteyn & Chopra, 2021).

For MCAS, hormonal shifts in pregnancy might modulate mast cell activity in ways we don't yet fully understand. There's early speculation that placental hormones may stabilize mast cells in some women, while others experience flares triggered by heightened immune sensitivity. These patterns could help identify subtypes of MCAS with different hormonal responses — but only if enough data is collected.

The role of patient registries and collaborative projects

A major change is happening with the creation of dedicated registries for pregnant patients with dysautonomia, connective tissue disorders, and mast cell diseases. These databases, often run in partnership with patient organizations, collect standardized information on symptoms, treatments, birth outcomes, and postpartum recovery. Over time, this will help identify patterns and guide treatment protocols.

The 2024 expert guideline project on managing pregnancy in hypermobile EDS and Hypermobility Spectrum Disorder is a good example. It's bringing together obstetricians, geneticists, rheumatologists, and patient advocates to create unified care pathways. This type of collaboration wasn't happening a decade ago, and it signals a growing recognition that women with these conditions deserve specific guidance, not just generic reassurance.

Where technology could change the game

Technology is starting to offer tools that can make care safer and more responsive. Wearable devices — already used by many POTS patients to monitor heart rate and activity — could be adapted for pregnancy monitoring, alerting providers to early signs of complications. Continuous blood pressure tracking might help catch hypotensive episodes before they cause a fainting spell.

In MCAS, future home-based biomarker testing could help identify triggers in real time, making it easier to adjust medication before a severe reaction occurs. And in EDS, imaging technology could improve detection of cervical or pelvic floor weakness before it leads to complications in labor.

Future therapies on the horizon

Several research teams are exploring treatments that could directly address the underlying biology of these conditions:

- **For MCAS**: more targeted mast cell stabilizers with fewer side effects than current options.

- **For EDS**: drugs aimed at improving collagen structure or signaling, potentially reducing tissue fragility.

- **For POTS**: therapies that regulate blood volume expansion without excessive salt intake or intravenous infusions.

If even one of these areas produces a safe, pregnancy-compatible treatment, the impact could be immediate and life-changing.

Why patient voices are reshaping the research agenda

The acceleration in research isn't just because scientists woke up one day and decided these conditions matter. It's because patients — mostly women — refused to be silent. They've built online communities, conducted informal surveys, and approached researchers directly with proposals. Organizations like Standing Up to POTS, The Ehlers-Danlos Society, and Mast Cell Action have used this energy to push for conferences, funding, and education campaigns aimed at obstetric and gynecological care providers.

This bottom-up pressure works. Specialists who used to dismiss POTS as "just anxiety" are now presenting at women's health conferences. Hospitals are starting to include connective tissue and autonomic disorders in their high-risk pregnancy guidelines. And as more women share their lived experiences, the cultural shift is making it harder for any clinician to ignore them.

Practical ways to stay connected to new developments

If you're living with POTS, EDS, or MCAS and want to keep up with the research without wading through endless journal articles, here's how to do it effectively:

1. **Join patient registries** — Your data helps build the evidence base, and you'll often get updates on findings.
2. **Follow reputable patient organizations** — Many publish plain-language summaries of new studies.
3. **Set up alerts for key medical journals** — You can filter for search terms like "pregnancy AND dysautonomia" or "Ehlers-Danlos AND obstetrics."
4. **Attend webinars or conferences** — Even virtual attendance can give you direct access to the latest findings.
5. **Work with your doctors to adapt new knowledge** — Bring printed summaries of relevant research to appointments.

The changing picture of care

The future is far from perfect, but it's no longer hopeless. Ten years ago, a pregnant woman with POTS might have been told to just "drink more water" and hope for the best. Today, she has access to individualized hydration protocols, labor position recommendations to reduce fainting risk, and postpartum plans for reintroducing medications.

In EDS, new obstetric protocols are addressing safe positioning during delivery to avoid joint injury. In MCAS, allergists are beginning to collaborate with obstetric teams to prepare emergency medication plans in advance of labor.

This change is uneven and still too dependent on patient self-advocacy — but it shows what's possible when awareness and research progress align.

Closing perspective – Building on the momentum

The real hope lies in keeping the momentum going. That means more funding, more collaboration, and more women speaking up about their needs. The research gaps are still wide, but the progress of the last few years proves that persistence works.

A future where no woman with POTS, EDS, or MCAS has to face pregnancy or menopause in fear is within reach. The more we contribute to the data, educate providers, and connect with each other, the closer we get. This isn't a fantasy — it's a slow, steady build toward a better standard of care.

Key takeaways

- POTS and EDS research in pregnancy is expanding, with generally positive outcome data.
- MCAS in pregnancy remains severely under-studied, but advocacy is pushing for change.
- Hormonal and circulatory changes explain some, but not all, symptom differences in pregnancy.
- Patient registries are essential for filling data gaps and guiding future protocols.
- Technology and targeted therapies hold real potential for improving care.
- Advocacy by women living with these conditions is driving the research agenda forward.

Appendix A – Symptom Tracker Templates

Tracking patterns is one of the fastest ways to help both you and your healthcare team see connections that might otherwise be missed. These printable templates are designed for long-term use and can be kept in a binder or as digital spreadsheets.

Menstrual Cycle Symptom Tracker

Track symptoms daily over at least three months to spot hormonal influences.

How to Use:

1. Write the cycle day at the top (Day 1 = first day of bleeding).
2. Record symptoms using severity scores (0 = none, 10 = worst imaginable).
3. Mark any changes in medications, diet, or stress.

Columns to Include:

- Date
- Cycle Day
- Symptom Ratings (e.g., dizziness, fatigue, abdominal pain, flushing, joint pain)
- Notes (new stressor, travel, illness)

Evidence Base: Symptom diaries improve detection of cyclic symptom patterns in POTS and MCAS, which often flare in the luteal phase (Raj et al., 2020)

Pregnancy Week-by-Week Symptom Tracker

Helps monitor trends and identify pregnancy-related changes that might require intervention.

How to Use:

- Start at Week 4 (when most pregnancies are detected) and continue through Week 40.
- Note vital signs (blood pressure, heart rate), hydration, symptom severity, and any medication changes.
- Bring this to every prenatal appointment.

Columns to Include:

- Pregnancy Week
- HR (morning/afternoon)
- BP (morning/afternoon)
- Main Symptoms
- Medication Changes
- Fetal Movement Notes

Evidence Base: Tracking vital signs during pregnancy in POTS helps detect orthostatic intolerance progression and preeclampsia earlier (Morgan et al., 2022)

Mast Cell Trigger Diary

Designed to pinpoint triggers for MCAS flare-ups.

How to Use:

- Record every food, beverage, medication, environmental exposure, and symptom onset time.
- Look for patterns after at least four weeks of consistent logging.

Columns to Include:

- Date/Time

- Intake/Exposure
- Symptom Onset (time after exposure)
- Symptom Type and Severity
- Relief Measures Taken

Evidence Base: Food-symptom diaries can reveal delayed hypersensitivity patterns not found in allergy testing (Castells et al., 2019)

Appendix B – Checklists and Worksheets

Pre-Pregnancy Planning Checklist for POTS/EDS/MCAS

Use before trying to conceive.

- Schedule a preconception consult with both your specialist and OB.
- Review all current medications for pregnancy safety.
- Update vaccinations.
- Optimize iron, vitamin D, and B12 levels.
- Create a flare management plan for pregnancy.
- Identify a delivery hospital with familiarity in dysautonomia and connective tissue disorders.

Hospital Bag Checklist for Chronic Illness

Pack at 35–36 weeks.

Medical Essentials:

- Medication supply (labeled, in original bottles)
- Compression stockings
- Electrolyte drinks
- Written medication and allergy list
- Mobility aids

Comfort & Symptom Control:

- Neck pillow
- Eye mask and earplugs
- Cooling towel

- Snacks safe for MCAS

Evidence Base: Hospital admissions are smoother when chronic illness patients bring self-management tools (Freeman et al., 2018).

Postpartum Recovery Checklist

Focuses on minimizing flares after birth.

- Arrange home help for first two weeks.
- Keep hydration and high-salt snacks at bedside.
- Use mobility aids if needed.
- Track bleeding, heart rate, and temperature daily for two weeks.

Care Planning Worksheet

Helps organize your personal management plan.

Sections to Complete:

- Diagnosis summary
- Current medications
- Allergies/intolerances
- Emergency contacts
- Preferred hospital
- Symptom flare protocol

Appendix C – Medication Safety Quick Reference

This quick reference lists prescription and over-the-counter drugs commonly used for symptom control in POTS, EDS, and MCAS. It is intended for patient education and should not replace medical advice. Always confirm any medication decision with your prescribing clinician, especially during pregnancy or breastfeeding.

Blood Volume and Blood Pressure Support

1. Fludrocortisone (Florinef)

- **Primary use**: Increases blood volume by helping the kidneys retain sodium and water; often used in POTS with low blood pressure.

- **Pregnancy safety**: Limited human data; animal studies show risk at high doses. Often considered if benefits outweigh risks.

- **Breastfeeding**: Unknown excretion in breast milk; monitor infant for fluid retention.

- **Special notes**: May require increased potassium intake to avoid low potassium levels. Alternatives include increased salt and fluids or compression garments.

2. Midodrine (ProAmatine)

- **Primary use**: Raises blood pressure by constricting blood vessels; used for orthostatic hypotension in POTS.

- **Pregnancy safety**: Limited human data; potential fetal risks; usually avoided unless essential.

- **Breastfeeding**: Unknown; generally avoided.

- **Special notes**: Taken during daytime only to avoid supine hypertension.

3. Droxidopa (Northera)

- **Primary use**: Increases blood pressure and may improve standing tolerance.
- **Pregnancy safety**: Insufficient data; avoid unless benefit outweighs risk.
- **Breastfeeding**: Unknown; monitor infant if used.
- **Special notes**: May cause headache or nausea.

Heart Rate Control

4. Beta-blockers (Propranolol, Metoprolol)

- **Primary use**: Reduce heart rate and palpitations in POTS.
- **Pregnancy safety**: Some agents (e.g., labetalol) used safely in pregnancy; propranolol/metoprolol generally considered with caution.
- **Breastfeeding**: Pass into breast milk; propranolol generally preferred due to short half-life.
- **Special notes**: Monitor for low blood pressure or fatigue.

5. Ivabradine (Corlanor)

- **Primary use**: Lowers heart rate without affecting blood pressure.
- **Pregnancy safety**: Contraindicated; teratogenic in animals.
- **Breastfeeding**: Avoid; no human data.
- **Special notes**: Only used in severe cases under strict supervision.

Salt and Fluid Retention Support

6. Oral rehydration solutions (e.g., Pedialyte, WHO ORS)

- **Primary use**: Maintain hydration and electrolyte balance in POTS.
- **Pregnancy safety**: Safe.
- **Breastfeeding**: Safe.
- **Special notes**: Look for low-sugar formulas to avoid spikes in blood sugar.

7. Sodium chloride tablets

- **Primary use**: Increase blood volume for POTS.
- **Pregnancy safety**: Generally safe if kidney function normal.
- **Breastfeeding**: Safe.
- **Special notes**: May worsen swelling in EDS-related venous issues.

Mast Cell Stabilization

8. Cromolyn sodium (Gastrocrom)

- **Primary use**: Stabilizes mast cells to reduce allergic-type reactions in MCAS.
- **Pregnancy safety**: Limited data; considered low risk as not systemically absorbed.
- **Breastfeeding**: Likely safe.
- **Special notes**: Often taken before meals.

9. Ketotifen

- **Primary use**: Mast cell stabilizer and antihistamine.
- **Pregnancy safety**: Limited data; avoid unless necessary.
- **Breastfeeding**: Unknown; caution advised.
- **Special notes**: May cause drowsiness.

Antihistamines

10. H1 blockers (Cetirizine, Loratadine, Fexofenadine)

- **Primary use**: Reduce histamine-related symptoms in MCAS.
- **Pregnancy safety**: Cetirizine and loratadine often preferred in pregnancy.
- **Breastfeeding**: Generally safe in standard doses.
- **Special notes**: Non-sedating agents preferred for daytime use.

11. H2 blockers (Famotidine)

- **Primary use**: Reduce stomach acid and help control MCAS symptoms.
- **Pregnancy safety**: Famotidine considered safe.
- **Breastfeeding**: Safe.
- **Special notes**: May be combined with H1 blockers for better control.

Pain and Symptom Control

12. Acetaminophen (Paracetamol)

- **Primary use**: Pain relief and fever reduction.
- **Pregnancy safety**: Safe at recommended doses; avoid long-term high use.
- **Breastfeeding**: Safe.
- **Special notes**: Avoid exceeding daily maximum dose.

13. NSAIDs (Ibuprofen, Naproxen)

- **Primary use**: Pain and inflammation relief; sometimes for EDS joint pain.

- **Pregnancy safety**: Avoid in third trimester due to risk of premature ductus arteriosus closure.
- **Breastfeeding**: Ibuprofen preferred; minimal transfer to milk.
- **Special notes**: Take with food to reduce stomach irritation.

14. Tramadol

- **Primary use**: Moderate pain control.
- **Pregnancy safety**: Avoid unless absolutely necessary.
- **Breastfeeding**: Avoid due to risk of infant sedation or respiratory depression.
- **Special notes**: Risk of dependence.

15. Low-dose naltrexone (LDN)

- **Primary use**: Off-label for pain modulation in EDS and MCAS inflammation.
- **Pregnancy safety**: Insufficient data; avoid unless benefit outweighs risk.
- **Breastfeeding**: Unknown; use with caution.
- **Special notes**: Must be compounded at low doses.

Other Symptom Management

16. Pyridostigmine (Mestinon)

- **Primary use**: Improves nerve signal transmission; can help POTS symptoms.
- **Pregnancy safety**: Used safely in myasthenia gravis during pregnancy; likely safe in POTS.
- **Breastfeeding**: Safe.
- **Special notes**: May cause stomach upset.

17. Ondansetron (Zofran)

- **Primary use**: Nausea control, especially in POTS with GI involvement.
- **Pregnancy safety**: Mixed data; often used when benefits outweigh risks.
- **Breastfeeding**: Likely safe.
- **Special notes**: Monitor for constipation.

18. Montelukast (Singulair)

- **Primary use**: Leukotriene receptor blocker; used in MCAS for airway symptoms.
- **Pregnancy safety**: Generally considered safe.
- **Breastfeeding**: Safe.
- **Special notes**: Monitor mood changes.

19. Hydroxyzine

- **Primary use**: Sedating antihistamine for MCAS flares and anxiety.
- **Pregnancy safety**: Avoid in first trimester if possible.
- **Breastfeeding**: May cause sedation in infant.
- **Special notes**: Can also be used short-term for sleep issues.

20. Aspirin (Low-dose)

- **Primary use**: Sometimes prescribed for clotting risk in certain EDS cases.
- **Pregnancy safety**: Low-dose may be used for preeclampsia prevention under medical supervision.
- **Breastfeeding**: Avoid high doses; low-dose under supervision may be safe.

- **Special notes**: Avoid in children due to Reye's syndrome risk.

Appendix D – Resources

Key Organizations

- **Standing Up to POTS** – Patient education and research funding.
- **The Ehlers-Danlos Society** – Global patient advocacy and medical education.
- **Mast Cell Disease Society** – Resources and physician directories.
- **Dysautonomia International** – Annual conferences and research grants.

Specialist Directories

- Ehlers-Danlos Society's physician directory.
- Dysautonomia International provider list.
- MCAS patient-led doctor database.

Suggested Reading

- Peer-reviewed guidelines on POTS management in pregnancy.
- Research on hEDS pregnancy outcomes.
- Reviews on mast cell disorders and reproductive health.

Evidence Base: Linking patients with condition-specific networks improves both disease knowledge and emotional well-being (Hoffman et al., 2020) (51).

References

1. Afrin, L. B., & Dempsey, T. T. (2019). Successful mast-cell–targeted treatment of chronic gynecologic pain and bleeding in five patients. Gynecological Endocrinology, 35(10), 844–848.

2. Afrin, L. B., Butterfield, J. H., Raithel, M., & Molderings, G. J. (2017). Often seen, rarely recognized: Mast cell activation disease — a guide to diagnosis and therapeutic options. Annals of Medicine, 48(3), 190–201.

3. American College of Obstetricians and Gynecologists (ACOG). (2019). Screening and management of bleeding disorders in adolescents with heavy menstrual bleeding. Obstetrics & Gynecology, 134(3), e71–e83.

4. American College of Obstetricians and Gynecologists (ACOG). (2020). Gynecologic considerations for adolescents and young women with cardiac conditions (including dysautonomia). Committee Opinion.

5. American College of Obstetricians and Gynecologists (ACOG). (2022). General approaches to medical management of menstrual suppression. Clinical Consensus.

6. Andrade, C., et al. (2021). Fludrocortisone use in pregnancy. Journal of Clinical Psychopharmacology, 41(1), 98–101.

7. Andrade, S. E., et al. (2021). Medication safety in pregnancy: Meta-analysis of registry data. Drug Safety, 44(3), 307–321.

8. Anjum, I., Ahmed, S., Aedma, K. K., & Ishaque, S. (2018). Postural orthostatic tachycardia syndrome and its management. Cureus, 10(8), e3125.

9. Arnold, A. C., Ng, J., Raj, S. R., & Fedorowski, A. (2018). Postural tachycardia syndrome. Autonomic Neuroscience, 215, 1–8.

10. Avis, N. E., Crawford, S. L., & Greendale, G. (2015). Duration of menopausal vasomotor symptoms over the menopause transition. JAMA Internal Medicine, 175(4), 531–539.

11. Aziz, Q. (2025). AGA clinical practice update on GI manifestations and autonomic or immune dysfunction in hypermobile Ehlers–Danlos syndrome. Clinical Gastroenterology and Hepatology. Advance online publication.

12. Blagowidow, N. (2020). Women's health concerns in Ehlers–Danlos syndromes and hypermobility spectrum disorders. The Ehlers-Danlos Society.

13. Blagowidow, N. (2021). Obstetrics and gynecology in Ehlers–Danlos syndromes. American Journal of Medical Genetics Part C: Seminars in Medical Genetics, 187(4), 581–588.

14. Blagowidow, N. (2021). Obstetric anesthesia considerations in Ehlers–Danlos syndromes. American Journal of Medical Genetics Part C: Seminars in Medical Genetics, 187(4), 589–596.

15. Blitshteyn, S., & Chopra, P. (2021). Hormonal influences on postural orthostatic tachycardia syndrome: Clinical observations and proposed mechanisms. Autonomic Neuroscience, 235, 102872.

16. Bourne, K. M., Chew, D. S., Stiles, L. E., et al. (2021). Symptom presentation and access to medical care in patients with postural orthostatic tachycardia syndrome. Frontiers in Neuroscience, 15, 724596.

17. Castells, M., et al. (2019). Food-related mast cell activation disorders. Journal of Allergy and Clinical Immunology: In Practice, 7(4), 1232–1239.

18. Christiansen, P., et al. (2020). Hormone replacement therapy in connective tissue disorders. Maturitas, 133, 16–23.

19. Ciach, K., Niedoszytko, M., Abacjew-Chmylko, A., et al. (2016). Pregnancy and delivery in patients with mastocytosis treated at the Polish Center of Excellence. PLOS ONE, 11(1), e0146924.

20. Demmler, J. C., Atkinson, M. D., Reinhold, E. J., Choy, E., Lyons, R. A., & Brophy, S. T. (2019). Diagnosed prevalence of Ehlers–Danlos syndrome and hypermobility spectrum disorder in Wales, UK. BMJ Open, 9(11), e031365.

21. Doherty, T. A., et al. (2018). Postural orthostatic tachycardia syndrome and the potential role of mast cells. Autonomic Neuroscience, 215, 83–88.

22. Dorff, S. R. (2020). Mast cell activation syndrome in pregnancy, delivery, postpartum and lactation: A narrative review. Immunology and Allergy Clinics of North America.

23. Dorff, S. R., & Afrin, L. B. (2020). Mast cell activation syndrome in pregnancy, delivery, postpartum, and lactation: A narrative review. Journal of Obstetrics and Gynaecology, 40(7), 889–901.

24. Dorff, S., Tinkle, B., & Levy, H. P. (2021). Obstetric outcomes in women with hypermobile Ehlers–Danlos syndrome. American Journal of Obstetrics & Gynecology MFM, 3(6), 100469.

25. Dukic, J., et al. (2024). Estradiol and progesterone from pregnancy to postpartum: fluctuations and implications. Global Women's Health, 4, Article 1428494.

26. Dysautonomia International. (n.d.). Postural orthostatic tachycardia syndrome.

27. Ehlers-Danlos Society. (2023). Menopause symptom survey results. Ehlers-Danlos Society Clinical Data Report.

28. Freeman, R., et al. (2018). Self-management strategies in dysautonomia. Clinical Autonomic Research, 28(1), 3–8.

29. Fu, Q., Vangundy, T. B., Shibata, S., Auchus, R. J., Williams, G. H., & Levine, B. D. (2010). Exercise training versus propranolol

in the treatment of the postural orthostatic tachycardia syndrome. Hypertension, 56(6), 1210–1216.

30. Fu, Q., Vangundy, T. B., Shibata, S., Auchus, R. J., Williams, G. H., & Levine, B. D. (2010). Menstrual cycle affects renal–adrenal and hemodynamic responses during prolonged standing in the postural orthostatic tachycardia syndrome. Hypertension, 56(1), 82–90.

31. Fu, Q., Vangundy, T. B., Shibata, S., Auchus, R. J., Williams, G. H., & Levine, B. D. (2018). Exercise training versus propranolol in the treatment of the postural orthostatic tachycardia syndrome. Hypertension, 72(1), 46–55.

32. Ghaith, S., Demmler, J., & Tinkle, B. T. (2023). Obstetric management of women with hypermobile Ehlers–Danlos syndrome and Hypermobility Spectrum Disorder. American Journal of Obstetrics & Gynecology MFM, 5(2), 100721.

33. Gilliam, E., et al. (2019). Urogenital and pelvic complications in EDS/HSD: A scoping review. Clinical Genetics, 97(1), 143–154.

34. Goff, A., et al. (2022). Menstrual cycle variability in symptoms of postural orthostatic tachycardia syndrome. Heart, Lung and Circulation, 31(Suppl. 2), S222.

35. Gülen, T., Hägglund, H., Sander, B., et al. (2021). Selecting the right criteria and proper classification to diagnose mast cell activation syndrome. The Journal of Allergy and Clinical Immunology: In Practice, 9(11), 4141–4148.

36. Guo, H., et al. (2023). Levonorgestrel IUD use in an adolescent with vascular EDS: A case report. Journal of Pediatric and Adolescent Gynecology, 36(2), 167–170.

37. Hagen, S., & Stark, D. (2011). Conservative prevention and management of pelvic organ prolapse in women. Cochrane Database of Systematic Reviews, 12, CD003882.

38. Hakim, A., et al. (2024). Hypermobile Ehlers-Danlos syndrome. GeneReviews.

39. Hoffman, S., et al. (2020). Patient-led networks in rare disease care. Orphanet Journal of Rare Diseases, 15, 183.

40. Hugon-Rodin, J., Lebègue, G., Becourt, S., Hamonet, C., & Gompel, A. (2016). Gynecologic symptoms and the influence on reproductive life in 386 women with hypermobility type Ehlers–Danlos syndrome: A cohort study. Orphanet Journal of Rare Diseases, 11, 124.

41. Hull, J., & Gilligan, L. (2018). Postpartum hemorrhage in connective tissue disorders: risks and management. Obstetric and Gynecologic Research, 2(1), 45–50.

42. Hurst, B. S., Lange, S. S., Kohn, J. R., & Markham, S. M. (2014). Obstetric and gynecologic challenges in women with Ehlers–Danlos syndrome. American Journal of Medical Genetics Part A, 164(2), 300–305.

43. International Federation of Gynecology and Obstetrics (FIGO). (2023). Uterine atony and uterotonics in postpartum haemorrhage. Statement.

44. Jensen, F., et al. (2010). Estradiol and progesterone regulate mast-cell migration and degranulation in the uterus. PLOS ONE, 5(12), e14409.

45. Källén, B., et al. (2013). Antihistamines during pregnancy. European Journal of Clinical Pharmacology, 69(5), 1163–1170.

46. Kanjwal, K. K., Karabin, B. L., Kanjwal, Y., & Grubb, B. P. (2009). Outcomes of pregnancy in patients with preexisting postural tachycardia syndrome. Pacing and Clinical Electrophysiology, 32(8), 1000–1003.

47. Kemp, S., Clegg, P. D., & Adams, S. B. (2018). Hypermobility and musculoskeletal pain in Ehlers-Danlos syndrome. BMJ, 362, k3036.

48. Kimpinski, K., Iodice, V., Sandroni, P., Low, P. A., & Fealey, R. D. (2010). Effect of pregnancy on postural tachycardia syndrome. Mayo Clinic Proceedings, 85(7), 639–644.

49. Kingsberg, S. A., et al. (2017). Vulvar and vaginal atrophy in postmenopausal women: findings from the REVIVE survey. Journal of Sexual Medicine, 14(4), 413–424.

50. Kohrt, W. M., Bloomfield, S. A., Little, K. D., et al. (2004). Physical activity and bone health. Medicine & Science in Sports & Exercise, 36(11), 1985–1996.

51. Kucharik, A. H., & Chang, C. (2020). The relationship between hypermobile Ehlers–Danlos syndrome, POTS, and MCAS. Clinical Reviews in Allergy & Immunology, 58(3), 273–297.

52. Kulas Søborg, M. L., Leganger, J., Rosenberg, J., & Burcharth, J. (2017). Establishment and baseline characteristics of a nationwide Danish Ehlers–Danlos syndrome cohort. Rheumatology, 56(5), 763–767.

53. Lei, D., Rapeport, G., & Goldust, M. (2017). Management of mastocytosis in pregnancy: A review. International Journal of Women's Dermatology, 3(3), 130–134.

54. Mackey, E., et al. (2022). Sex differences in mast cell–associated disorders. Cold Spring Harbor Perspectives in Medicine, 14(10), a039172.

55. Malfait, F., Francomano, C., Byers, P., et al. (2017). The 2017 international classification of the Ehlers–Danlos syndromes. American Journal of Medical Genetics Part C: Seminars in Medical Genetics, 175(1), 8–26.

56. Mast Cell Action. (2021, September 13). Mast cell activation syndrome in pregnancy: Guidance for obstetric providers.

57. Miller, A. J., Stiles, L. E., Sheehan, T., et al. (2020). Prevalence of hypermobile Ehlers–Danlos syndrome in postural

orthostatic tachycardia syndrome. Autonomic Neuroscience, 224, 102637.

58. Molderings, G. J., Brettner, S., Homann, J., & Afrin, L. B. (2016). Pharmacological treatment options for mast cell activation disease. Naunyn-Schmiedeberg's Archives of Pharmacology, 389, 671–694.

59. Molderings, G. J., Brettner, S., & Homann, J. (2020). Mast cell activation disease and pregnancy: Current knowledge and future directions. Journal of Obstetric Medicine, 13(4), 221–229.

60. Monaco, A., et al. (2022). Association of mast-cell–related conditions with hypermobile EDS. American Journal of Medical Genetics Part C: Seminars in Medical Genetics, 190(2), 211–221.

61. Morgan, A., White, P., & Smith, R. (2022). Pregnancy outcomes in women with postural orthostatic tachycardia syndrome. BJOG: An International Journal of Obstetrics & Gynaecology, 129(5), 851–859.

62. Morgan, K., et al. (2022). Orthostatic intolerance and pregnancy outcomes. American Journal of Obstetrics & Gynecology, 227(3), 384.e1–384.e9.

63. Morgan, K., Smith, A., & Blitshteyn, S. (2022). POTS and pregnancy: Review and recommendations. International Journal of Women's Health, 14, 1831–1847.

64. Morgan, K., Wickson-Griffiths, A., & Kanjwal, K. (2022). POTS and pregnancy: A review of literature and recommendations for evaluation and treatment. International Journal of Women's Health, 14, 1435–1449.

65. Narita, S. I., et al. (2007). Environmental estrogens induce mast cell degranulation and enhance IgE-mediated release of

allergic mediators. Environmental Health Perspectives, 115(1), 48–52.

66. National Center for Advancing Translational Sciences. (2022). Patient advocacy resources. U.S. Department of Health and Human Services.

67. Nunez-Pellot, C., et al. (2025). Lactation safety of cardiovascular medications. Breastfeeding Medicine, 20(1), 15–22.

68. Özdemir, Ö., et al. (2024). Mast cell activation syndrome: An up-to-date review. Allergy, Asthma & Clinical Immunology, 20, 21.

69. Pearce, G., Bell, L., Pezaro, S., & Reinhold, E. (2023). Childbearing with hypermobile Ehlers–Danlos syndrome and hypermobility spectrum disorders: A large international survey of outcomes and complications. International Journal of Environmental Research and Public Health, 20(20), 6957.

70. Peggs, K. J., Nguyen, H., Enayat, D., Keller, N. R., Al-Hendy, A., & Raj, S. R. (2012). Gynecologic disorders and menstrual cycle lightheadedness in postural tachycardia syndrome. International Journal of Gynecology & Obstetrics, 118(3), 242–246.

71. Pezaro, S., et al. (2024). Management of childbearing with hypermobile Ehlers–Danlos syndrome and hypermobility spectrum disorders: A scoping review and expert co-creation of evidence-based clinical guidelines. PLOS ONE, 19(5), e0302401.

72. Raj, S. R. (2013). Postural tachycardia syndrome (POTS). Circulation, 127(23), 2336–2342.

73. Raj, S. R., Black, B. K., Biaggioni, I., Paranjape, S. Y., Ramirez, M., Dupont, W. D., & Robertson, D. (2009). Propranolol decreases tachycardia and improves symptoms in the postural

tachycardia syndrome: Less is more. Circulation, 120(9), 725–734.

74. Raj, S. R., Fedorowski, A., & Sheldon, R. S. (2022). Diagnosis and management of postural orthostatic tachycardia syndrome. CMAJ, 194(10), E378–E385.

75. Raj, S. R., Guzman, J. C., Harvey, P., et al. (2020). Canadian Cardiovascular Society position statement on postural orthostatic tachycardia syndrome (POTS) and related disorders of chronic orthostatic intolerance. Canadian Journal of Cardiology, 36(3), 357–372.

76. Raj, S. R., et al. (2020). Menstrual cycle influences on postural tachycardia syndrome symptoms. Autonomic Neuroscience, 228, 102717.

77. Raj, S. R., Guzman, J. C., Harvey, P., & Vernino, S. (2022). Multidisciplinary management of postural tachycardia syndrome. Autonomic Neuroscience, 237, 102930.

78. Roux, C., Briot, K., & Horlait, S. (2016). Bone loss after menopause: diagnosis and prevention. Climacteric, 19(5), 397–404.

79. Ruzieh, M., Grubb, B., & Karabin, B. (2018). Overview of the management of postural tachycardia syndrome in pregnancy. Autonomic Neuroscience: Basic and Clinical, 215, 63–66.

80. Sheldon, R. S., Grubb, B. P., Olshansky, B., et al. (2015). 2015 Heart Rhythm Society expert consensus statement on the diagnosis and treatment of postural tachycardia syndrome, inappropriate sinus tachycardia, and vasovagal syncope. Heart Rhythm, 12(6), e41–e63.

81. So, D., et al. (2010). Safety of antihistamines during pregnancy and lactation. Journal of Allergy and Clinical Immunology, 125(2), 619–623.

82. Standing Up to POTS. (2023, June 20). Gynecological issues & pregnancy in MCAS with Dr. Shanda Dorff.

83. Standing Up to POTS. (2023). Living with POTS: Patient and clinician resources. Standing Up to POTS.

84. Standing Up to POTS. (2024). POTS cheat sheet for healthcare practitioners.

85. Stickford, A. S. L., VanGundy, T. B., Levine, B. D., & Fu, Q. (2015). Menstrual cycle phase does not affect sympathetic neural activity but modulates blood pressure and vasoconstriction in women with POTS. Frontiers in Physiology, 6, 28.

86. Stiles, L. E., Cinnamon, J., & Moralez, G. (2018). What POTS patients wish their doctors knew. Autonomic Neuroscience, 215, 121–122.

87. Stuenkel, C. A., et al. (2015). Treatment of symptoms of the menopause: an Endocrine Society clinical practice guideline. Journal of Clinical Endocrinology & Metabolism, 100(11), 3975–4011.

88. Tai, F. W. D., Palsson, O. S., Lam, C. Y., et al. (2020). Functional gastrointestinal disorders are increased in joint hypermobility–related disorders with concomitant POTS. Neurogastroenterology & Motility, 32(12), e13975.

89. The Ehlers-Danlos Society. (2024, May 30). Management of childbearing with hypermobile Ehlers-Danlos syndrome and hypermobility spectrum disorders (news summary).

90. Thompson, J. M., et al. (2020). Acetaminophen and developmental outcomes. Pediatrics, 146(1), e20194162.

91. Wang, X., et al. (2018). Menopause and autonomic function changes. Menopause, 25(10), 1131–1138.

92. Weiler, C. R., Butterfield, J., Binstadt, B., et al. (2020). Mast cell activation syndrome: Tools for diagnosis and differential diagnosis. The Journal of Allergy and Clinical Immunology: In Practice, 8(2), 498–506.

93. Woidacki, K., Meyer, N., Schumacher, A., Goldschmidt, A., Maurer, M., & Zenclussen, A. C. (2014). Relevance of mast cells in pregnancy. Clinical Reviews in Allergy & Immunology, 46(2), 124–134.

94. World Health Organization. (2023). Endometriosis: Fact sheet.

95. Wu, F. C., Tajar, A., Pye, S. R., et al. (2010). Hypothalamic-pituitary-testicular axis disruptions in older men are linked to ill health. Journal of Clinical Endocrinology & Metabolism, 95(8), 3838–3846.

96. Wu, X., et al. (2025). Effects of postpartum hormonal changes on immune system dynamics. Acta Biochimica Polonica.

97. Yaşa, C., & Sandal, K. (2020). Approach to abnormal uterine bleeding in adolescents. Turkish Archives of Pediatrics, 55(Suppl 1), S3–S10.

98. Zaitsu, M., et al. (2007). Estradiol activates mast cells via a non-genomic estrogen receptor-mediated pathway. Cellular Signalling, 19(1), 7–19.

99. Zhao, S., Tran, H., & Tan, J. (2023). Postural orthostatic tachycardia syndrome. In StatPearls. StatPearls Publishing.

www.ingramcontent.com/pod-product-compliance
Lightning Source LLC
Chambersburg PA
CBHW070243100426
42743CB00011B/2110